The Whiskey Journal:

Definitely Not a NATO Role III MMU Publication

C.W. Rastall

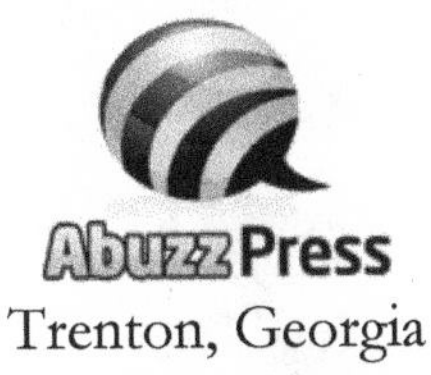

Trenton, Georgia

Print ISBN: 978-1-64719-855-8
Ebook ISBN: 978-1-64719-856-5

Library of Congress Cataloging in Publication Data
Rastall, C.W.
The Whiskey Journal: Definitely Not a NATO Role III MMU Publication by C.W. Rastall
Library of Congress Control Number: 2021920069

Published by Abuzz Press, Trenton, Georgia, U.S.A.

Printed on acid-free paper.

Abuzz Press
2022

Disclaimer:
The views expressed in this publication are those of the author and do not necessarily reflect the official policy or position of the Department of Defense or the U.S. government. The public release clearance of this publication by the Department of Defense does not imply Department of Defense endorsement or factual accuracy of the material.

Dedicated to:

A classy lady of many names, but most known to me as

Grandma Mongin

Table of Contents

Introduction .... **- 1 -**

Part I: Getting There .... **- 5 -**

PROLOGUE .... - 7 -

THE SECOND CLASS ASSOCIATION .... - 17 -

MY FATHER AND THE NAVY .... - 31 -

GRINDR .... - 41 -

ME AND THE CAP'N MAKING IT HAPPEN .... - 47 -

DR. CHRISTINA "DEAREST" SOLOMON .... - 61 -

SPADES .... - 81 -

PRISON GYM .... - 95 -

Part II: Arrival .... **- 105 -**

LETTERS FROM HOME .... - 115 -

JESSE JOHN .... - 163 -

THE PHARMACIST .... - 187 -

ICU NURSES .... - 217 -

FITZ .... - 231 -

THE THIRSTY CAMEL .... - 241 -

THE BRASS .... - 257 -

FREDDIE .... - 273 -

Part III: Coming Home .... **- 275 -**

Afterword .... **- 311 -**

Stillness Is the Key Inscriptions .... **- 315 -**

Introduction

If you are the reader that is looking for the blood and glory of war, this is not the right book for you. Within these pages there is no wild shoot-out or dramatic moment that can easily make its way onto the pages of a screenplay. This is not a story fit for the movies or the thrill seekers of imagination. No, this is a story of what happens when all that is removed, and you have just a man with his thoughts.

What started as an intention to keep a historical record of my time while serving in the United States Navy's longest running overseas combat hospital, and its last rotation at that, this project morphed into something more. For the 231 days I was gone, from the days I kissed my family goodbye at the Fukuoka, Japan, International Airport, to the day I rolled up and surprised them at home, I wrote a page for every single day of my deployment as a Sailor in Whiskey Rotation for the NATO Role III Multinational Medical Unit hospital.

These pages that follow serve as little reminders of what I endured, sacrificed, and learned while underway. It was written in a time when COVID started out as just a joke but ended with one of the most abrupt welcome-home transitions ever. Yes, COVID, that invisible force of destruction which altered so much of the world I had left behind. It rocked the deployment and robbed me of many opportunities that so many others were able to cherish. I started my journey when it started its warpath, and when I came home, it still lingered into the fabric of a culture I find hard to now recognize.

So, what is interesting about this book? It is a story about the journey of a Sailor on their first deployment. From a firsthand experience, the trials and triumphs are examined. From start to finish, the character arc is established, built, and finished. The same person did not return to the same place they started. Think of it as a boy becomes a man, or the ugly duckling becomes the beautiful swan. This is a book of transformation through the experiences in the environment. In this case, it was in Kandahar, Afghanistan.

My origins are humble enough. I was raised in suburbia Wisconsin and joined the Navy after flunking out of a small University of Wisconsin school. I had a lackluster Navy career thus far; there was nothing remarkable about my life except that I knew that I had something within me, a story that could be told. This feeling compounded when I saw the marketplace of forgettable but still-published content from armed service veterans. I am not a Navy SEAL, and I don't have a coffee company, but I refuse to marginalize my experiences and accept that they have something more worthy to say than me.

Please enjoy and appreciate the journey as I have. There were so many people that I met and learned from. A friend once told me that although writing is a linear product, it is a cyclical process. I'll need to take her word for it; she does after all have a doctorate degree in literature. My original intent was to transcribe my journal word-for-word, find the easiest way to reprint and publish in an eBook format, and share with my friends and family. If only the road less taken was the easier path.

I noticed many problems in my journals and shifted rudders multiple times to rechart the course. People, places, and things may have been obvious to me, but were not likely familiar to the wider audience. I took for granted the importance of character development, and why anyone should care as much as I did about the people I chose to write about. Lastly, upon my own review and the guiding hand of mentors, it very quickly became apparent that some of my feelings were written in haste with a narrow scope of empathy toward some people. This of course had to be revisited, and there were tweaks made to paint as many people as I could with the dignified character I have grown to admire about them in hindsight. With that established, I don't always say the nicest things, and hopefully it was written with the intent of establishing a baseline and the reader can read about the growth of my relationship with them. Everything has been revised to a PG-13 rating. Although Grandma knows how Sailors talk, it does not mean she wants to read it in a complete and unabridged copy.

In no way am I out to divulge Navy secrets or tarnish the reputation of the service I currently serve. In fact, this memoir is just the opposite of that juicy tell-all. It's a daily account of my life while deployed and honors those I served with. It took me years to realize just how much of a team we are all on, not only the Navy, but the Armed Forces as a whole. Me pushing ibuprofen in Japan has a butterfly effect with the boots on the ground in operational theaters. If anything, I write about the aspects of a deployment that aren't harrowing fear, arduous bloodshed, or selfless glory. It's the opinion of this author that most deployments align with what I am about to share.

Here is a quick summary of what I left behind. My wife of nine years, Saori, who was three months pregnant with our third child, unknown to us yet another boy. My oldest son Josiah, who was four when I left. His first little brother Atticus, who was two. Separately, they are nicknamed Josey, after the outlaw Josey Wales, and Atti, because he had not gone to law school. Together when "the boys" are referenced, it is because I am referring to them. I was stationed in Sasebo, Japan, and, upholding the highest traditions and values of Japanese culture, my divorced mother-in-law, Miyuki, was our roommate. Or maybe I was the tenant, because we call our home the house Saori grew up in as a child. Because I was given 5% of the house for paperwork reasons, I do like to brag that I am a homeowner now, but I digress.

Miyuki is as tough as they come. In December 2016 she was diagnosed with stage 3 pancreatic cancer. Although I had what we call "verbal" orders to Naval Hospital Yokosuka, through bureaucracy and the guiding hand of an army of guardian angels, my tour was rerouted to Sasebo upon leaving Branch Health Clinic Iwakuni, Japan, in February 2017. The intent was to be stationed closer to home so Miyuki could ride off in a familiar place. As this is written, she refuses to die, teaching me nothing less than what grit, perseverance, and determination looks like when it's personified. She might love Japan more than I love Wisconsin, and I love her all the more for it.

Alas, this has been a transcription from two 5" x 10" journals. What does this mean exactly? Sometimes what I have to say is brief, and I restricted myself from flexing literary tools used for structure. It was my goal to remain as true to the primary text as possible, but it is my hope to fill in enough of the picture to provide an entertaining story of my journey with the attachment of a postscript after each entry and a supporting substory sprinkled throughout the text.

Part I:
Getting There

PROLOGUE

That August day in 2019 started like any other. I drove into work bored, frustrated, and burnt-out. Hardly the winning combination for the makings of a success story, but there I was enjoying another fine Navy day. At the time I didn't have much going for me except for the realization that I would be slugging out another one and half more years at Naval Branch Health Clinic Sasebo for a nearly unprecedented five years. Since checking into the command in April 2017, there was nothing conventional about my time there. Then again there was nothing conventional about my time in the Navy to begin with.

April 2017 was the mark of the beginning of my end. I was entering my second duty station as a Second Class Petty Officer, or the rank of E-5, and was growing long in the tooth when it came to being promoted. I remembered when I first came into the Navy back in 2008 and heard the stories of career-serving Sailors retiring at 20 years as an E-3. By my generation, that era had long come to pass, and it was almost mythical to see a retiree's ID card saying they were anything less than an E-6. Due to a retention program called High Year Tenure, or HYT, the Navy, because I can't speak for the other armed service branches, set restrictions on service past a certain year provided you were not a specific rank or above. In 2017, that magic number was 14 years or you prepared to perform the seabag drag on a one-way ticket back home. There I was into my 11th year.

It was fine though, I had it all mapped out. I was only a handful of classes from graduating with two bachelor's degrees that I felt were diversified enough to get my foot in the door across a spectrum of platforms no matter how entry-level they were. I'd carry with me over a decade of military experiences, and I had a load of veteran benefits awaiting me on the other side. My family was young enough to survive the trauma of short-term unemployment and small enough to still crash in a basement of a family member back in Wisconsin until I could get back on my feet.

So, for the next three years, the original length of my assignment to Sasebo, I was going to pack it in, think of only myself, and prepare for the great transition back into the civilian workforce. There are plenty of successful people who make the leap and I was going to be one of them. It was easy for me to imagine being so selfish. I felt I was terribly wronged at my previous command when it came to evaluation rankings, so trying to please the boss was not going to be my first concern anymore. Those junior Sailors would survive without my presence just like the Navy did and will continue to do after I'm long out of the picture.

My plan had hiccups from the beginning though. The first problem was I was spiritually dead from not being a positive member to my community. Serving has always been my thing. My first intended major at the University of Wisconsin - Green Bay was public administration because I wanted to be part of public service. To willfully retract my involvement and talent from my community caused a downward spiral in my mind. This feeling did not take long to drag my soul down to a very low place. It wasn't until a friend of mine, Petty Officer Matt Crosson, called me from my previous duty station and asked me to pin him to the next higher paygrade that I decided to change. He had recently been promoted and thought high enough of the impact I had on his life to request I make the journey to "frock" him to my current paygrade, E-5. This was the same guy who I first met as a lowly E-3, so to see his journey was a real joy.

The second problem was a fact of life. We uphold the highest traditions and customs in my home, aptly named Camp Rastall, or NAVCOMCMPRSTL, and that includes a multigenerational home. Since we were back living in Japan and Saori, my wife, had a divorced mother, she started living with us in 2014. The concept of a mother-in-law living with them could make any American husband cringe with anxiety, but for the most part it really worked out. Miyuki, or "Okasan," helped with the household chores, and when we added onto the family, starting with our first-born Josiah in 2015, it mattered a great deal that she was with us. It was all good until the stomach pain started.

It was the winter of 2016, and Miyuki started getting terrible stomach pains. The first doctor brushed off the worst symptoms. Pain management is almost non-existent in Japan. My wife had a cesarean section with our child, was given an indomethacin suppository, and told to lay still. Indomethacin is a non-steroidal anti-inflammatory drug, or NSAID, which is in the same drug class as ibuprofen. The pain in Okasan's stomach would not go away, and eventually she went to another doctor where she was diagnosed with stage 3 pancreatic cancer in December. This is the same cancer that took Patrick Swayze and Alex Trebeck. To have this condition means you have less than a 5% chance of living past five years. The countdown was on.

At the same time, I received verbal orders to Naval Hospital Yokosuka, Japan. A little farther north from where I was in Marine Corps Air Station Iwakuni, Japan, (both on the same island of Honshu) but it was in the opposite direction from Sasebo, Japan, (on the southern island of Kyushu) and where Saori was from. To compound the situation, Saori was pregnant with our second son, Atticus. With all the news, Miyuki made the decision that she wanted to move back to the home where she raised her family to essentially die. My wife, not one to leave her mother, told me this and went on to explain that she wasn't going to abandon her mother. It was presented to me that I could head up to Yokosuka without my wife, two-year-old son, dying mother-in-law, and unborn child, or I could try to find a way to come back to Sasebo, my first-ever duty station that I served at from 2009 to 2011.

Despite these setbacks both personally and professionally, I had made up my mind that I wanted to put care and effort into my career. Miyuki's good health lingered longer than any of us expected, and I realized that I had to extend my stay in Sasebo to care for her. One extension turned into two, and that is when I received the text message. It was from my co-worker Yanara Lopez, who did nothing except excel at everything she did. To be fair, she paid the price for it in terms of ridiculous working hours and exhaustion, but she could flat outperform anyone else. Because I decided to be difficult so early in my tour, (we had arrived about a week apart from one another) I spent the better part of three years hanging onto her coattails. We had always been amicable, and when she asked me if I wanted to go to Afghanistan, it changed the trajectory of my life probably forever.

I remember parking my car, doing my daily routine to prepare for the morning, and then heading straight into our Senior Enlisted Leader's (SEL) office, Master Chief Lorenzo Branch. I let him know that I heard the rumor about a pharmacy technician being needed to go to

Afghanistan, and if the rumor was true to please consider me for the shortlist. Master Chief has a talent I do not have. He can show an excellent poker face, and to this day I can't figure out what he may have been thinking at that time. My hope is he appreciated the initiative and enthusiasm to chase "the hard job." What he did was simply tell me that he'd let me know.

Fast forward to Labor Day weekend, I get a phone call from him to formally ask me if I wanted to accept the deployment. Because it was just me going and not a unit, it is called an "Individual Augmentee" or IA. Without hesitation I leapt at the chance. This was my chance to deploy, and not just anywhere, but to Afghanistan at the longest-serving Navy combat hospital. What lies next is my journey from the day I left to the day I returned home. Every day wasn't easy, but I was blessed more than many others if only for the fact that I came home at all to write about it.

17 Feb 2020
Day 1

As I write this, I am at the Narita Airport awaiting my flight to Dallas/Ft. Worth on American Airlines Flight 176. I left not one but two Leatherman multi-tools in my carry-on. This was a result of hastily packing the night before against my wife's superior judgment. Needless to say, airport security in Fukuoka had some questions for me, and I was last to board on my flight to Tokyo while $200 worth of multi-tools stayed behind.

There were a few really good going away dinners and parties. This past Saturday I went out to the bars and took my first ever beer bong, and it was worth my troubles. Jack Adams and Dennis Lebling, who were there, are two friends I hope to know for a long time.

The hardest part in all of this was saying goodbye to the boys. Because of time, we were rushed to begin with, but the tears started coming the farther in the security line I was. The levees broke when I was almost to the security counter and I heard Josey yell, "Bye Papa!" That was much harder than I ever anticipated.

Of course, I did not accomplish every goal I had, and I doubt I would have anyway. There's never enough time. Prior to leaving I found it hard for me to concentrate, and I often became lost in fits of daydreaming. Normally, I'm trying to think about problems and solving them in my head as far as my imagination or logic will allow.

I hope to sleep a lot on the plane. Will write more when I can and I'm thankful to Kevin Pham for this journal. I suppose I'll be transcribing too.

Postscript: No amount of time would have prepared me to leave. I was first given the greenlight for this deployment on Labor Day weekend, 2019, and on the day I was at the airport, I still felt hurried and rushed. Perhaps that is human nature, but to me it showed the reality that although your own life is getting tossed upside down, everyone else around you is still trying to run their own race and get through the struggles of their own day.

17 Feb 2020
Via Facebook Messenger

Hey buddy,
I miss you. Thank you for all the lessons you've taught me and I'm grateful for all the lessons we've learned together. I appreciate you always having my back and being someone I can vent to; in many ways you were like an older brother-uncle hybrid and you've guided me seamlessly through some obstacles. I'm glad we've been able to laugh and create memories that I'll be telling my kids about; like how I lifted a piano, one-handed, onto an 8ft-tall truck bed, and their Great-Uncle Cal was there recording (unfortunately the film got lost over the years, haha). Your absence will be truly felt, not just at home by your wife and two little munchkins, but for the little folk like me who just happened to have orders to Sasebo. I love you buddy, and I hope over the years to come we always stay in touch.
Yours to count on,
Travon [Martin]

18 Feb 2020
Day 2

Yesterday was the longest day of my life. Although the flight to Dallas took only 10.5 hours as opposed to the normal 12 to Chicago, they placed me at the windowless emergency exit seat. It did not matter how much leg room I had because I couldn't fully sit back. I spent the flight hunched forward. It was bad. On top of that it was an American flight crew, and the Asian airlines rule the skies. There are times I'm not interested in experience.

My hotel is nice. I do enjoy the Holiday Inn Express variety. The car rental is a Volkswagen Jetta. Nice car, but I need to relearn American/Virginian driving. Had a Samsung Galaxy Smartwatch delivered to the hotel. As I write this, it is being paired now.

Met the pharmacy crew today. Spent the most time with LCDR Vince Deguzman. He asks a lot of questions, and they are plain enough to where I must constantly check myself for military bearing and statesmanship. No doubt he's being polite, but first impressions matter. The other two First Classes, Jacob Wilson and Michael LePenna, remain to be assumed about.

I personally am talking more with the E-4s & below, but tomorrow will make more of an effort to get to know the other E-5s. Still too early to figure out who the alpha is, but I am not lacking in my own confidence. Jet lag was "fine" today, but the real test will be the next 2-3 days.

Postscript: There were several days that could be thought of as the longest of my life. Even when those days happened, I need to remember that I lived through them, and at worst they will be the tinder for a good story. The first couple of days that the Whiskey Rotation came together were really a bunch of mini-interviews, and it was necessary to build the relationships we needed to have for the next several months. A brief lesson on ranks: I am an E-5, and there are nine enlisted ranks starting at E-1. There are 10 officer ranks, and a LCDR, or O-4, is short for Lieutenant Commander in the Navy and Coast Guard. In every other branch it is called

"Major." Why the Navy chooses to be different is a question that might forever elude me.

21 Feb 2020
Days 3, 4 & 5

These past couple of days have blown by. As I predicted, the jet lag has been worse than Day 1. A typical day might have me getting back from work, sleeping until about 2300 or so, staying awake for a couple of hours, getting 90-120 minutes of napping, and I'm up again at 0430. Then I shower and putt around the room, and I'm out the door for sure by 0530 and I'm STILL caught in traffic.

The Norfolk-area highway still amazes me, I have never seen so many cops, broken down cars, and traffic. The Navy sure knows how to pick'em as I stand by my original feeling, that Norfolk and the Tidewater area is for the birds.

We were released early on Wednesday, and I visited our two main former residences: 50 Ireland St. and 130 Loch Circle, both of Hampton fame. Neither property looked occupied and honestly, they looked like they've seen better days. Maybe my eyes matured. Saori seemed appreciative when I took pictures.

Speaking of Saori, I need to try to get in a groove to talk to just her. Every time I call it's around mealtime, and it's just to coax the boys into eating. Not much time for the adults to talk.

I'm still working on getting the Second Classes to come together. Maybe because I am so much more senior/experienced remains to be seen, but I haven't found my friendly rival just yet.

They selected the most junior Role III Sailors to stand Auxiliary Security Force (ASF). In front of the Senior Enlisted Advisor (SEA), HMCS Cameron Wink, I told my Leading Petty Officer (LPO), HM1 Wilson, that I wanted to help write the watchbill and to add me to the ASF team.

I wish I could have taken a picture of their faces. I have nothing to lose and am going to commit myself.

I'd really like to find that one guy who can really push me again, the friendly rival. Matt Crosson is coming up from Camp Lejeune, North Carolina, tonight, supposedly for two days. It will be nice to see and discuss life with a familiar face.

Also, I think I am going to return my smart watch. It is irritating my skin more than a $300 watch should, and that is an unnecessary distraction. Today is Friday, and there was no work. Norfolk got about a 1/4 inch of snow, and everyone lost their minds. So, we finished processing yesterday and received today and tomorrow off.

I have spent my day doing laundry especially, but caved and bought clippers to manscape with. Target had no multi-purpose oil, so, sucks-to-be-me, I had to go to Home Depot. It did not disappoint. I will pack my first seabag and try to mail it back today. Hopefully they have Military Postal Service (MPS) benefits here.

Postscript: They did not have MPS service here as that is reserved for only overseas bases. Maybe I would have known that if a majority of my military career had not been overseas. The original intention was to write one page at the end of each day, but it turned into one page for each day. In other words, entries with multiple days were written all in one sitting, and it covered those days. Some minor details may have been missed when this happened, but it also allowed me space to write about other ideas and concepts running through my mind. It was very important to me to establish myself as a team player and as a performer. I carried with me a common proverb: "If you want to go fast, go alone. If you want to go far, go together."

23 Feb 2020
Days 6 & 7

As I write this, I am on a plane headed for Camp Pendleton, California. It's a military flight that left from the Oceana Naval Air Base, and because it was just the 80 or so of us, it was roomy in the cabin, but lacking many

amenities. To be fair, it lacked many rules too. I'm sure somewhere the Federal Aviation Administration has some oversight, but military flights are the definitive way to fly if given the choice.
The two days I spent with Crosson were much needed. It is fun to talk to him like a peer and not as a superior. We met when he was two ranks subordinate to me, but his intellect and determination have propelled him to my own rank. We collectively used our brains to create a great discussion. At first, I was a little concerned that we might run out of things to talk about or stay trapped in the mindless loop of only bonding with Iwakuni (Marine Corps Air Station Iwakuni, Japan) memories we had together. This was clearly not the case. Something tells me he would have said similar things if he kept a journal.

While waiting for our flight, I had my first real conversation with HM1 Wilson. So far, there's high stock on him. It's hard for me to articulate to him just how ready I want to be to leave it all out on the field and perform any way he picks. Maybe "needs" is a better word. This is a definite know-your-role and trust-your-chain-of-command type situation. To perform, inspire, lead, and follow. Because Crosson drove me to the airport, and we arrived not a moment too soon at the terminal, I was warmly greeted by some HM2s this morning. So, I will call that a start in the right direction.

Postscript: As fond as the memory with Crosson was, the conversation with Wilson was the paragraph that stole this entry. My intention was to not just establish rapport but also expectations and give him a sense of who his subordinate was. To my fortune, and as time would tell, he was an adaptive enough leader to recognize and understand the kind of Sailor and man he was talking to, but neither of us knew that at the time. He has said he pegged the kind of guy I was by our first email correspondence prior to meeting in Norfolk, and will have to believe him, but the most important take-away from that talk was, as the leader, he listened to what I had to say.

24 Feb 2020
Day 8

I'm very tired this evening. This place is nothing like I ever stayed at or experienced in the past. First of all, Camp Pendleton is huge, but our lodging is one upgrade up from a tent. It's open bay but with cots. I get a half-size trunk to put my things.

Luckily I slept like a lamb of God. Everyone else, not so much. Turns out my worst fear is confirmed; my snoring is a bit problematic. Someone said they think someone had apnea, and the logical guess is they were talking about me.

This week we are doing the exact same thing I was sent to Iwakuni for, TCCC (Tactical Combat Casualty Care)! As one might expect, I'm not very happy, but I have to roll with these punches. There is more inefficiency than I thought there'd be. If ever given the chance, I hope to constructively point some things out.

Called Saori today, and I noticed privacy here is harder to come by. I left my Sapphire mobile Wi-Fi brick on the bus, and this makes me upset and mad. There is a nurse talking on the phone in the same room I'm in, and it's entertaining me overhearing her problems. A lot of first-world problems.

Starting to make better friends with the HM2s and had a good dinner with pharmacist LCDR V. Deguzman.

Postscript: For someone who had never been to Camp Pendleton, California, such as myself, the compound we stayed at was pretty barren. Then again, in hindsight, I was privileged with a pretty cushy career so far. I have never been "greenside," or a Corpsman attached to a Marine unit. I never slept in the field or had to dig a hole for a toilet. The compound actually had Wi-Fi throughout the area. The sleep apnea part was maybe me, but some of us were notorious snorers. I am proud to join their ranks.

THE SECOND CLASS ASSOCIATION

Whiskey Rotation had 20 Second Class Petty Officers in total. All except one, our pay officer, was a Hospital Corpsman. Like any peer group I was closer to some than others, but as a whole, I loved them more than the whole damn bunch put together. Being a Second Class, or PO2, is an interesting place to be because you're not junior enough to get the brunt end of the work no one wants to do, but you're also not senior enough to be the first person yelled at by the Chiefs. It's a rank normally called the best in the enlisted force. The problem for me is that I had overstayed my welcome as a "deuce," and it was beginning to show.

Like any promotion, you must work into the new role and gradually expand your abilities and therefore extend your credibility with leadership. There is a grace period that is unsaid yet understood in shedding off the habits and expectations of the rank inferior to the one you now wear. Then there is a turning point, one where you ripen in your rank and start to assume roles that the next rank would typically carry. This was me, and what I wanted to do most of all was somehow showcase that I'd done all that I could as a Second Class and would be an ideal candidate to transition into the next higher pay grade. Many of my frustrations were built on the fact I was not yet a First Class Petty Officer, and it was that glass ceiling that spawned so much conflict throughout so many relationships.

This did not deter me from what I loved to do most, team-building and committee work. Someone long ago once shared with me that the hardest thing anyone will ever do in their professional job is lead their peers. I considered this my final frontier as a Second Class and wanted to quickly establish a good rapport with my cohorts while building a committee, which required us to unite and tackle projects bigger than any one of us could perform had we been solo. These peer-leadership groups have different names depending on the rank you are in.

For the most junior Sailors, there is the Junior Enlisted Association, or JEA, and this generally covers E-1 to E-4. Because the idea is Second Classes will replace their "big brothers and sisters," and we want to emulate them, there is the Second Class Petty Officer Association (SCPOA) and First Class Petty Officer Association (FCPOA). Senior enlisted, the Chiefs, have something that we call "the Mess" or "Goat Locker." Sounds funny, but ask anyone and it's the Mess that keeps the Navy humming along.

Creating an SCPOA was an ideal challenge for me by grabbing the largest rank of the deployment together and generating a cohesive unit despite being whipped together from literally over the world. Although we never officially got it going with bylaws and elections, I think I had a role in applying a gel that kept us together despite our numbers and diversity. It was also not some coy power play to establish dominance. To me, it was a necessary task that needed to happen, and without anyone saying anything to me, I attempted to set it in motion. Even without an official organization, it had an important value to me from a very early stage in the deployment as I wanted to be a part of leading my peers.

It's because of this interest in government, so to speak, that I developed a couple of nicknames throughout my peer group(s), which include "The Governor" and "Judge." I accept those monikers with pride and tried to uphold the namesakes. After all, my dream job is to one day become the governor of Wisconsin. How can I lead a state if I can't lead a bunch of E-5s? Ever since third grade when I was elected by my class to become their Student Council representative at Richmond Elementary School, home of the Rockets (Appleton, WI), a purpose of public service began to grow inside of me. Besides running for class secretary in 10th grade, I have never run for anything besides the president of any peer organization.

As President Bartlett told Josh Lyman in *The West Wing* (1999): "You want to know the difference between Leo [his Chief of Staff] and me? I want to be the guy, and Leo wants to be the guy who the guy depends on." For every Steve Jobs, there needs to be a Steve Wozniak. For every leader who thinks up and out, there has to be a leader who dives down and in. This creates balance, and any social group needs both to perform optimally. Although I am more of a President Bartlett, I understand that there are Leo's out there, and they must be given their proper respect and room to create their best work. I think this comes with time, experience, and maturity. All of those words may sound synonymous, and in some circles they are, but I treat them differently. Identifying what the team needs most is a skill, and a way to sharpen that skill is to throw yourself into the fires of failure.

Another way is by reading and reading and then reading some more. The importance of expanding your knowledge base cannot be understated, and it is accomplished by propping yourself up on the shoulders of giants. Although it's now a cliche, it is true that leaders are readers, and if you're not entering every day starving with curiosity, when the time comes when you are expected to know the answer, do not be surprised if you come up short. To me a book is still the ultimate tool in reading, but I can also use the term loosely by expanding to audiobooks as well. Instead of listening to the radio on my drive into work, why not quench my thirst for more knowledge. This does not marginalize fiction either, which has its importance. Fiction exercises the mind too and generates creativity and self-exploration. Lastly, using "YouTube University" to learn something you didn't know before through visual learning has exponential benefits too.

Some days I become very mad at myself for not being promoted. There is no one else to blame except me. I could shake my fist at the world, but it's certainly too busy to give me special consideration. While I'm stuck here though, I'm making the most of my time and being as productive as possible. One day the call will come, and until then I need to continue aligning my words with my actions. That starts with going to work, being a professional, trying my hardest, and doing things for the right reasons. When the day comes to work HM1 out of a job, I want to be ready because it's the least I can do and in the best interest of those who I'm expected to serve.

The deployment may not have forged these ideas, but they certainly solidified them. So, in that regard, I'm thankful I was able to go on that journey with 19 other very decent human beings and it was our progress that we accomplished together that helped make the deployment so enriching not only to my career, but to my soul.

25 Feb 2020
Day 9

I've started to keep the day number on top of my pages. Hopefully, it will make me happier than sad. Called the boys at around 0730 Japan time. Atticus seems much more interested in seeing me than Josiah. He appears to be more inconvenienced than anything, but this could possibly be his way of projecting his grief. Either way, I really think Saori is going to erase the YouTube app from the Amazon Fire Stick though, and I don't blame her.

I'm extra tired today, and that might be because I did some "exercise" this morning. In reality I went for a walk down the road and listened to my audiobook. Still working on Chernow's *Grant.* By the time I returned, my calves were sore. It really is almost pathetic. Baby steps into it though. Today I only ate galley food, which I would think is a step in the right direction.

Today was just classroom stuff, but I did see HMC Geiger. He was HM2 Geiger back in 2010 the first time I was stationed in Sasebo. Kristoph Carey and I had a good chuckle and caught up a little bit on Messenger.

Currently fishing for a roommate. First two casts came up short. Who knows, maybe I'll get my own room. Unlikely. Tomorrow we test out, again.

Postscript: There are better written books by more accomplished authors who have touched on their journey through weight loss. Although it's touched on multiple times throughout these pages, the physical fitness journey was only a pixel in the whole picture. This does not take away the fact that being in the armed services should require and demand an expectation of not being sore from just walking. It was a long road, but some life lessons had not yet been pounded into me.

26 Feb 2020
Day 10

What a day. For it being a half day, I was finished with TCCC by 0940, and there seems to be plenty to say. First of all, today is my 12-year birthday in the Navy. This one seems a little more special than others to me. Slight pay increase, gold stripes, and 8 years until retirement, provided I can promote at least one more time. It's also my brother Maxwell's birthday, but more importantly it's his 21st. I sent a meme on the family group chat, but besides that I have been silently keeping his safety in my thoughts this day.

Our class has been released for overnight liberty should we choose to take it. Well, I don't know anyone well enough or at all to justify leaving the compound here. Saved some money eating at the galley, but all of this was done alone. Called my parents and we talked for about 12 minutes. Will most likely call Rich later. When I called Saori, it just seemed like I was competing for her attention. Because I think that's a little messed up, the talk didn't last long.

Bought a notebook and envelopes so I might just write a letter, but to who or when remains a mystery. I think, in conclusion, it still doesn't feel like I'm deployed and "gone." Listening to Tool now to feel a little closer.

Postscript: Closer to what you might say? Closer to feeling back in my comfort zone. Many Sailors were stationed in the San Diego/Camp Pendleton area, so this liberty was very important to them. Maybe part of me wanted to begin my misery of the deployment as soon as possible, and that meant seeking isolation from everything that I love and know. Anyone's 21st birthday always spooks me. Although it's probably not their first time at the rodeo, I'm still concerned for their decision-making. My 21st birthday was essentially a week-long festival. I had just graduated from Hospital Corps School a week prior and my beak was rather dry. Luckily, I had the best friends in Green Bay who I still cherish to this day.

27 Feb 2020
Day 11

As I write, it is technically the 28th, but early enough in my day to write with clarity of yesterday. We had liberty all day, but instead of sleeping in, I was up at 0530 to take HM3 [Redacted] to his Physical Screening Test (PST) for his Force Reconnaissance Corpsman "C" school. As it turns out, the pool opened at 1000, not 0700. In that case, we went to have an All-American breakfast at Denny's. It was awesome, but not the best. Waffle House with Matt Crosson was better, but HM3 [Redacted] is such an interesting guy to talk to.

After returning to the compound, I was snatched up by three other HM2s. We ended up at Barnes & Noble where I lost my damn mind. I dropped $125 on books and fell short at my goal of picking up a Spanish copy of *Twilight* for my good friend Jenna Fitcher (Smith). They were out of stock. Maybe in Texas a book 15 years old will be popular.

After the bookstore, we dropped off the rental vans that had been issued to the unit, and that took forever. Upon our arrival we cleaned the compound, from sweeping the floors to cleaning the bathrooms. Then came the best part of the entire trip, Gabe Hansen picked me up. It was so delightful seeing him again and catching up. We found a local Mexican place and I had the long-anticipated California burrito. I think it was worth the hype, and it was a solid recommendation from Matt Crosson. After we parted ways, I finally began laundry until I couldn't keep my eyes open. It was 2215.

Postscript: Throughout the text the time is written in the military fashion. There is no way around this; it is too ingrained in me. If you get confused, just subtract 12 hours from anything after 1300 and that is the time. My dinner with Gabe should not have been downplayed. This was a chucklehead I worked with in Sasebo. He was not only a solid and go-to worker for the Sconnie Sailor Moving Company (more on that later) but became my friend. I was very happy to know and see him.

29 Feb 2020
Day 12 and 13

Welcome to El Paso, Texas. More to the point, I have been told that I'm technically in New Mexico. If that is true, I can add one more state I've never been to. Well, sort of. I'm not allowed to leave the base, but nor would I want to.

I'm starting to get into a battle rhythm, or at least the skeleton of one. Enough of all that introduction jazz because I have some things to get off my chest, and I have two pages to do it. More times than not, when I write, I'll have YouTube's Critical Drinker accent in my mind. Leaving Camp Pendleton was a happy experience because I did not like or appreciate the Naval Expeditionary Medical Training Center's rules or living conditions. Yes, great to see Opie (HN Gabe Hansen) again, and eat at a Marine Corps galley, but that's the end of my list.

Seeing the Sailors from the San Diego area with their wives and girlfriends only reminded me of how I was so bad at saying goodbye to my own family, and how I'm going to regret that for a long time.

Somehow, someway, the flight from San Diego to El Paso was an hour. Although I was asleep for most of it, what I did see from the Texan air was one from another planet. I keep find myself asking "where the hell are we" with each new stop. Nothing but flat. In the horizon there is mountains-ish, I guess. Crosson was right, everything here or close to Mexico takes on a yellowish hue like in the movies. I can't think of a more boring or basic place in the United States.

Technically I'm located on the McGregor Range in Las Cruces, New Mexico. The barracks are old, smelly, and borderline criminal. I volunteered to be the Supply Petty Officer. I have access to my own room because it is doubling as the storage closet. The job has that one ginormous perk. Senior Chief Wink knows about it and has willed it. Just can't mess up the job now.

Today is leap day, and I started intermittent fasting by cutting out dinner. I like breakfast too much. So far so good, except I will eventually need to get more disciplined on the carb intake. More on my thoughts as we progress. I also started PT-ing twice a day. I woke up at 0445 and headed to the track. Didn't get very far. Did the same thing in the evening. Same result, felt marginally better, but the wind sucked. Tomorrow I will try and build from it.

Postscript: This will not be my first time talking about what life in Texas was like. I do know that being the Supply Petty Officer was a double-edged sword. I had my own room, yes, and not even the Commanding Officer had that luxury by the time our trip to Texas was over. On the other hand, it made me incredibly popular with anything facility and supply related. It made for some interesting times, but I think I made the most of the opportunity. For example, I was able to meet everyone, and I was never out of toilet paper, which was a pretty big deal this time of year.

1 Mar 2020
Day 14

Today was rather uneventful. Went to the gym after calling the boys. They are so much more agreeable right before they go to bed. At the gym I climbed on the treadmill...and it wasn't good. At a speed of 4.5 mph, I only lasted 10 minutes without stopping. Closed out the 30-minute run at 2 mph. I know, not good. I then did some foam rolling, which felt good, yet painful.

Showered at the gym even though I forgot my shower shoes in my room. Then forgot my Common Access Card (CAC) for breakfast. Made it to muster on time, then slept. Woke up for lunch, then slept some more. I did a load of laundry and finally sat down to read my Laura Ingalls Wilder biography. That's one thing I am noticing, and it's starting to really chap my ass that I am placing YouTube as a higher priority than my books and actual progressive goals. I should only be able to watch so many film theory critiques or intermittent fasting videos.

Speaking of, day two in Texas is coming to a close. Big breakfast and lunch, no bubble gum after lunch. After laundry, I called Saori. I begin to see how stressed she's becoming because of Miyuki's prognosis. After that I walked 3 miles around the 0.6-mile track, or 5 laps. Just walked. Maybe I'm sick?

Postscript: It is more important to me to mark one's failures than successes. They will serve as a reminder and benchmark for where improvement is most needed. If you're not your own worst critic, then don't count on anyone else offering to give you the hard news. Miyuki is my wife's mother, and up until this point has been battling with pancreatic cancer. Although it's a bad joke, she refuses to die, and if there is anyone who has taught me about resiliency, grit, and determination, it's her.

2 Mar 2020
Day 15

It's hard to believe it's only been two weeks. Then again, I'm not sure what to exactly think of it. Still so recent, yet so far away from Saori and the boys.

Today we picked up the beginning of what we call CIF, or Combat Issue Facility, I think. Just chest plates, helmet, and maybe some other stuff. Honestly, I wasn't exactly paying close attention today, just going with the flow and getting through the day. This base (Fort Bliss) is nothing memorable except that it's so boring. The food is bland, the land is flat, and now I know what Anakin Skywalker was talking about with his dislike for sand in *Episode II*.

I did however splurge for Chipotle. In fact, I lost my damn mind eating both a bowl and a burrito. Like that wasn't enough, I then waddled to Dairy Queen where I had a cookie dough with Reese's blizzard. Amazing.

The part of the day after lunch was the best because a few PO2s and I really started gelling, I think. One of them even started to call me the President of the JEA (Junior Enlisted Association). It was flattering, and hopefully it sticks.

Showed some improvement on the treadmill today. Went 4.5 mph speed but lasted 15 minutes without stopping. Feeling jazzed.

Postscript: Wisconsin has its problems, but one is not the scenery. If you look past the farmers' fields, there is in fact a lot to stare at. Japan is a splendid visual display of color, mostly green, or at least the part of the country I live in. Texas I'm sure is a diverse place, but we begin dipping into my disgust for this part of America. I'd rather live in Chicago. Also being a proud Wisconsinite, I do not understand why Dairy Queen exists in the state anymore ever since it became "Culver's Country." Still, DQ brings me back to my most youthful days.

3 Mar 2020
Day 15

So, I'm entering this submission a little early because I don't feel like wasting any time packing it in this evening after muster. It was actually raining today, and I find that very surprising because, to be honest, I didn't think I would personally ever see it rain in the desert. Maybe strange around some water coolers and funny among some campfires, but it's probably my ignorance talking most likely.

We are in the Army now. All three of our classes today were Army-specific and did not include medical, Role III, or the Navy. One brief was about convoys. Somehow this lecture was spread across two hours. The lecturer started his "brief" by saying that he's been in for 23 years, recently divorced with no more kids, so it's just him and the Army these days. Ouch. Hearing him talk, the guy's mind is still partially in one of his four Iraq tours. I'll leave it at that except I don't want to be him.

Went to the gym and under-performed. Only 10 minutes at 4.5 mph pace on the treadmill. I did clear yesterday's sins in the restroom though which was a relief. For some reason the cardio room was closed tonight so I didn't work out. Only ate one meal today to get back on track, and I handled it with grace.

Postscript: This lecturer, a Sergeant First Class, or Army E-7, stayed in our minds the entire tour. Only a few more notable characters along the journey left a more lasting impression, but to me it revealed some hard truths about warfare, Iraq and Afghanistan, and the damage left in its wake. Post-Traumatic Stress Disorder is a real thing, and this guy was the embodiment of this condition. I've seen it before with fellow Hospital Corpsmen attached to Marine units, and there is a lot of guilt that they lived while their Marines did not. Some keep it buried within a box in their mind that does not get shared, others discuss it openly to cope, but either way and across the spectrum, if you choose to engage, I cannot recommend enough that it be approached with a level of respect and dignity only found in the most noteworthy of circumstances.

6 Mar 2020
Day 16, 17 & 18

So, I'm clearly a couple days behind on this, but I can easily explain why. Simply enough, I was not in the right headspace to put anything on paper. Rather, I had to think out my problems, which I am now comfortable enough to share here.

Before that, I will say that I got my first piece of deployment mail today, and of course it was from my mother. It was very touching and I'm thankful I keep such mementos.

Yesterday I sent a slew of letters and postcards off, including the memory book for Grandma Mongin. I really hope it takes off and people actually write in it based on the questions in the book and the answers she provides. A huge regret I have, is that I am not there to do that project myself.

On a random thought, my mother did make a subtle recommendation to buy Dennis and Teresa's home if they were ever to move to Arizona. I think the idea demands pause for reflection because I am catching myself daydreaming about it. It's hard to be thinking of actually owning a home, but how far-fetched is the idea really? Will definitely be bringing this thought up again.

Back to life on an Army base. I think I've established how much I don't like it and how desolate this area in general is. How sad I get when I see rocks in a yard where there should be grass. Well, the training we are doing isn't much better. Lately, we have been learning about Improvised Explosive Devices, or IEDs, and pretty much every aspect of them. How this pertains to medicine and the Navy is beyond me, but once again we are obliging the good Commanding General's orders.

Honestly, it's hard to write about specifics for a couple of reasons. One, I'm not exactly paying attention because I'm trying to numb my mind, and two, this is all wasted time, and I'm doing what I can to pass that time.

Which brings me to the crux of my latest problem, my place in this deployment. I know in my heart I am doing something that matters. I am going into a combat zone. What I don't feel yet is a sense of self-importance. Lately I was getting bent out of shape over the HM1s getting all the looks for leadership roles. When do the Second Classes get their shot at proving their worth to lead?

I think my problem is that I'm losing sight of it being a marathon and not a sprint. We are only on day 18 so I can prove my worth by being the best teammate possible. I can lead by supporting and not causing any trouble. To be the best version of myself and to make each day my masterpiece.

Yesterday I did a good job on the treadmill, sort of. New modern record of 17:30 at 4.5 mph pace. One day I'm going to finish Chernow's *Grant*. It is not enjoyable anymore, and this leaves me caught up with entries!

Postscript: The feeling of "what is my role" is a haunting thought, and one that I've struggled with for as far back as I can remember. How badly I wanted this to be my Spanish-American war that Theodore Roosevelt had; a time of glory, a flex of my ability to handle and conquer what he had called "the strenuous life." When you are willing to charge your San Juan Hill, you don't want to consider the other elements critical to achieving organizational readiness. I was not burdened with having to organize and forge a unit that came straggling in from across the world. I did not have to answer the questions that would stump everyone else in the room. I did not have to acknowledge that there was more to leadership than what I was seeing from my perspective at the time. This feeling of incompetence and eagerness was a mark of immaturity of the mind despite being in the highest percentile in terms of years of service. Rank, Chain of Command, and hierarchy in general have their place in military theory, and although I was more than ready to buck the system, it was actually not going to be me to turn the institution on its head.

MY FATHER AND THE NAVY

I was born to Kim and Elly Rastall on a hot day in August 1987. Years later I was told that my conception was the result of a young wife not being able to wait and get upstairs to their apartment after her husband returned from a hunting trip in the northern Wisconsin woods the previous November. There is also another piece of family lore that I lived in that same apartment for only one day until we moved to Teluah Avenue in Appleton, Wisconsin. To me, Appleton is famous for two reasons: it is the city 40 miles away from Green Bay, WI, that has a hotel nice enough to host visiting teams that play the Packers, and it is home of the Harry Houdini Museum. Appleton was my first hometown though, and I am glad I was able to live there for the first 10 years of my life.

My father died in 1994 to leukemia. Although I was only six at the time of his passing, there are memories I still have and cherish. For the most part, my memory of him was mostly instilled in me by stories of the other people who knew him best. There is nothing wrong with that, but I think there are times when his legend gets hammed up a bit, but either way it does not make me smile any less about him. For the longest time I knew that he too was in the Navy, but there was really no one I could ask about it. Years later while serving onboard the USS Theodore Roosevelt (CVN 71), I was encouraged to petition the US National Archives for his military personnel file. So I did, and the first time they sent me his DD-214, or Certificate of Release of Discharge from Active Duty. All it said was he served for about a year and left the service without a single promotion, leaving as an E-1. So I petitioned again, and when I received his full service record, I understood why the National Archives may have been hesitant to release it to the man's eldest son.

Within a year, on just one ship, my father was sent to Captain's Mast, the Navy's version of non-judicial punishment under the Uniform Code of Military Justice, not once, but three times. His last notation was about a pending court martial. This was in the early 70s, and one of the things he was in trouble for was having marijuana in his bed. There were a couple of other times when he was charged with unauthorized absence, and he just didn't show up for work for days at a time. I cannot imagine being the legal officer, his immediate leadership, or ship's administrative department dealing with this hellcat. When I joined the Navy, I wanted to honor his legacy in a way, but he simply made it too easy for me.

From time to time I will take out his personnel file and bring it into work. A lot of the paperwork is much the same as it is today, so it's easy enough to translate to young Sailors. Not many people can believe that the son of the man they were reading about would one day write a book, and I am glad it was a windy day when the apple fell from the tree.

My father "recovered" from his misadventure in the Navy and landed a blue-collar job working in the paper mills of the Fox Valley area of Wisconsin. He married his first wife and that is how my big sister Rachael came into the world. Young marriages are hard to sustain, so when that ended a more seasoned and mature Kim John Rastall married the last daughter of Ambrose and Virginia Mongin, Elinor.

8 Mar 2020
Day 19 & 20

Yesterday was our field practicum for Improvised Explosive Device, or IED training. Like every other training so far it was stupid. They make us wear all this Kevlar and other Army crap like a helmet and vest with plates in. When we got out to the field, they realized we were not only all Navy, but medical and mostly reservists. This meant they essentially spoon-fed us the answers and made it as easy as possible, which in some circles was hard to believe because we were out there for 75 unbelievable minutes. When we returned, we sat around waiting for everyone else to finish.

Had a MRE (Meal Ready to Eat) for lunch and was walking back to the barracks by 1300. Did my travel claim; getting that behind me was maybe the only bright spot of my day. Then I realized the Wi-Fi was out across base, so I took a nap.

Woke up and then proceeded to plunder the Marine Corps Exchange (MCX) for absolute crap, but that wasn't the strangest part of my day because I went to the MWR lounge and tried to play a video game. It was on a PlayStation 4, and the game was Marvel vs. Capcom. The Chuck E. Cheese arcade model was infinitely better. Closed out the day by talking to my mom and hearing about Jonica and Arron.

Today was filled with some more wasted time. We went to the range today to shoot some shotguns with non-lethal shells. There was no qualifying, just familiarization of a weapon we are not issued and don't earn "credit" for learning. On top of that there was a little bit of rain and a cold wind across the desert. These games ended when the buses picked us up at 1145.

Then I went to Texas Roadhouse Steakhouse, again, with PS2 Robert Krombach and another Second Class. Had a few good laughs and parted ways shortly after. I went to see a movie. It was the new Ben Affleck flick, *The Way Back*. It was essentially *Hoosiers* 2.0 if Scooter was the coach instead, but it had its tear-jerking moments.

Also, today I applied for the Public Affairs Officer job. I got my copies of the *Sasebo Sun* and wrote a quick paragraph of my credentials. They will likely give it to an actual officer, but you never know and maybe I'll actually get to interview.

This weekend was stupid. I was undisciplined with my diet and PT (or lack thereof) and it's 2100 and I'm just now getting to do my laundry. Called Saori too.

Postscript: Within the Whiskey Rotation, there were reservists who were redeploying back to the Role III for a second time. For newbies like me, we hung onto their words like they were the gospel because we had to get a frame of reference from somewhere.

What they shared about the Role III hospital had me even more agitated that we were doing all of this stuff, but on the other hand, those veterans were the most chilled-out of everyone. They certainly rolled with the prerequisites to get into the combat theater, and understood it was just part of the process. The most frustrating part for me was simply not knowing how this game was played. My sister Jonica (for clarity my stepsister) was divorcing her husband, and I had feelings about that. Not only did I like Arron, but in my head, I think of the brothers-in-law of my mother's side of the family: Uncle Mike, Steve, and my dad. They are some of the most respected and oldest members of my family, and I always like seeing them interact with not only each other, but our family. They have been in the family for so long there is no distinguishment. I suppose I wanted that, but I also do not have Jonica's life.

11 Mar 2020
Day 21, 22, & 23

Pause for a moment of joy: when I called home this morning, the boys were getting ready for bed, and it was the first time I was able to see Atticus peeing standing up. Like so many of the boys' "first" moments, odds are this was nothing new to Saori, but it made me smile.

Although I'm not a fan of saving multiple days to write at once, it seems to be the trend. I was thinking about why, and I think it's because I don't have a table in my room. For example, it's 0800 on March 11 and I'm sitting in class "learning" about DAGR, or some sort of navigation system. Point is, there is a table and I'm using it for its purpose, to actually write on.

Two days ago, we simulated a Humvee rollover. It was cool in the sense that it broke the mold of traditional classroom learning. I closed my eyes and waited for it to be over like any amusement park roller coaster, then crawled out. The problem with all of this "training" is that there are no stakes, no tension, no consequences. We all pass, there is no measure of competency, no fear of failure. Therefore, why try or put in effort? Sometimes I wish I wasn't such a Debbie Downer, but cookie-cutter training is pointless. Also on Day 21, we learned basic radio operations. Should I ever have to get on the radio, it's going to mean we are having a really bad day. Day 21 was a full day but paled in comparison to Day 22.

Yesterday we were on the M9 gun range. It was a day of memories. Long story short, I had to qualify three times. There were 30 targets and I had to hit 16. The third time they loaded my magazines twice the correct amount. It was literally the worst kept secret. It was sunny after a cool morning and an hour-long bus ride which pushed off at 0645. We didn't return until 1600.

On the way home I was so tired I was drooling on myself. There was one goal in mind, and it was to finish the nap I had started on the bus in my bed. My uniform wasn't completely off yet, and people were already knocking on my door looking for gun cleaning kits. I got snippy in a hurry. Needless to say, I did not fall back asleep.

Then there is the peer pressure. They all mean well but come on man! HM1 Jacob Wilson invited me to go lift with him, and Krombach was giving me hell for getting some ice-cream at dinner. After two MRE's, it was nice to eat real food. Consequently, I am missing breakfast today, and to get back on track will need to miss dinner.

I also did jog on a treadmill for just 10 minutes before I had to crap. To be fair, my evening became a little busier. It came to my and everyone else's attention that I have been appointed as the Leading Petty Officer, or LPO of the Public Affairs Office team. There is a primary lead, Lieutenant Commander (LCDR) Kate Fitzgerald. Her deputy officer is Lieutenant (LT) Simon Prado. I was in a van with him once at Camp Pendleton, so not much else to say about him except he asked to read my copies of the *Sasebo Sun*. The rest of the team are enlisted and I'm the most senior. HM3 Ho Vo and HM3 "Bernie" will be our photographers. I specialize in writing and the newsletter aspect of the program. LCDR Fitz sounds like she wants to spearhead the Role III Cruise Book. Because we formed just last night, a lot remains to be seen, but I was dominating the WhatsApp conversation and narrative. Luckily, all the enlisted belong to the same directorate, so we are organizationally close for communication purposes.

I was thinking last night, and I'm positioned to be in a good place. If the MWR fund gets turned over to me, and I handle that cash, I will have a corner on the Junior Enlisted Association (JEA)/Hospital Corpsmen (HM) Ball, Morale Recreation and Welfare (MWR), Public Affair Office (PAO), and Pharmacy LPO. Oh, and we haven't even stepped foot in Afghanistan yet. My strategy will be to keep staying hungry and bringing all with me for the ride.

Postscript: Leadership is a universal concept. Good leaders can thrive in diverse environments. That is why we see many CEOs jump from one field to another. They are also everywhere on the spectrum. Some are mature and ready while others are budding and learning. They are at the highest levels of organizational charts and at the very bottom. Leaders will thrive in the environment they're in. With all of that said, leaders know how to count. They understand that certain roles provide other or more opportunities, and that there is usually a quantifiable number next to those roles when placed on an evaluation score sheet. Leaders are selfless, but also need to be pragmatic. They are not dumb, blind, or lame. Leaders hustle, grind, calculate, and sacrifice. This was also the introduction of the most exciting part of my job, the Public Affairs Office.

12 Mar 2020
Day 24

May this day be quickly forgotten except for what is said on this page. The day sucked, and there isn't any way to sugarcoat it. We start with a lazy morning. I did eat breakfast, however, a smart one at that. Everything else was tossed aside, such as shaving and showering. I just didn't care to get out of bed, and I know why.

Today we did land navigation, but it was the Boy Scout way with a map made of paper, metal compass, and a protractor. It was biblical. So, they "teach" us for two hours and then drop us in the middle of the desert. I was part of a team of seven, and we were supposed to find five targets. I think we found three. We walked in the desert like nomads. The only nice thing about it was we were in the foxhole together.

Upon limping back to the barracks, there were blistered feet to nurse. I walked to submit a trouble-ticket or two, then got some food from the MCX and YouTubed for a moment. Showered at the gym, and HM2 Wilbon Robinson got me some Buffalo Wild Wings.

The highlight of my day was talking to Saori, and she thought I looked like I've been losing weight. And so, it begins.

Postscript: Yes, so it began. As delightful as it was to hear from the missus, I wouldn't be able to measure any progress until we were actually in Afghanistan. I heard about a nurse having bought a scale, but I was too shy to ask to use it in case the reading did not give a good answer. The land navigation day really frustrated me, and I know I should have taken this time in El Paso as an opportunity to learn and think of it as an adventure, but that simply was not the case. It was a wall to slow me down from getting to the real mission where it really mattered.

13 Mar 2020
Day 25

Happy Friday the 13th. Oh boy, it did not disappoint. By far, this day was my least favorite day in Texas. It's hard to describe what I did, but I know I did it in the rain. We're talking about "swim qual" amounts. It was uncomfortable and I wasn't in the mood.

Didn't eat breakfast and got to Fort Bliss "Freedom Crossing" in time for lunch at 1300. Well, 1345 because it takes so long from Camp McGregor. Anyway, wrote a little to the Koontz family. Back to lunch today, I ate Chipotle. Just a burrito this time. I also ate a Cinnabon for the first time ever. The adventure was topped off when I boarded the bus with a Dairy Queen banana split for the first time in about 25 years. It was a mistake to eat it because it was not bringing back the memories of my youth. That's all I ate today. No food until lunch tomorrow.

Hopefully I can get back to only missing one meal. I miss breakfast. I'm writing from my bed. I think the handwriting is worse off than usual. I didn't nap today, but I didn't PT either. A lot of YouTube and I need to do some serious cleaning of my room. Plus, I need to get on the track.

Postscript: What we did was play patrol, and in a way that was the capstone of what we had learned so far. We were in our flack gear; I'm already immobile because I'm the fattest person in the unit, and it was not an exaggeration on the rain. There I was, with 20 other clueless medical professionals, trying to set up a perimeter because we think we see a landmine in the middle of the road. This was about every 30 feet or so, and the instructors finally told us there were no more for the rest of the exercise. It was a nice amalgam of dumb and embarrassing. I don't think I'll ever eat a Dairy Queen banana split again; it just didn't taste the same as the five-year-old me had remembered, and that disappointment will stick with a fellow for a long time.

15 Mar 2020
Day 26 & 27

It has been an interesting past couple of days, and today is not even over. I'm at the gun range waiting to be driven back to the barracks. We shot two other guns and the .50 caliber. It is definitely an assault rifle. Now that I shot it in person, I laugh that Alicia Keys was able to whip it around and through hotels during *Smoking Aces* in 2006. I always did like that movie more than I should.

Some other guys are playing music on a speaker. They're playing Mariah Carey's "We Belong Together" and my eyes are catching allergies. I think of Jim Hackett and a girl I used to know. I digress though as they are old memories. Not sure what else I'm going to do today. Probably start deciding what's going back to Japan or being forwarded to Kandahar.

Will also look into renting *Parasite* (2019). It won best picture so I should see what the commotion is all about. That said, I have yet to see last year's best picture *Green Book* (2018), which always seemed like *Driving Miss Daisy* (1989) but with dudes instead.

That leads me into what I watched last night. My oldest brother, Dylan, highly recommended *The Lighthouse* (2019) with Willem Dafoe and

Robert Pattinson. I was not ready. Clearly an artsy film, full of imagery and deeper meanings. I don't think I was in the mood to see it, but it passed a couple of hours.

Then there was the first real problem so far. The person behind my fake Grindr profile came back and started talking to members of the unit, again. At first it was flattering and humbling, but the fact it repeated, and it was obviously coming from within the unit, well, I made the unilateral decision to bring it up the chain of command. Started with HM1 Jacob Wilson and he heard my story attentively and with professionalism before disclosing he'll have to bring it to Chief. That night I told both Chief and Senior Chief. They were empathetic and said they'd address the enlisted. Not exactly the best way to head into a six-month deployment to Afghanistan.

Otherwise, it was a slow past couple of days, but that's the way she has been going. The boys are getting bigger and more addicted to TV. Atticus remains more interested in talking to me, but they both say "hi."

Postscript: Guns have little utility in my life. I recognize they have their purpose as both a practical tool to hunt and for self-defense, but I was never one to get excited for guns. There are those who wake up harder than Chinese algebra to shoot them and know everything about them. There isn't one photo of me, to my knowledge, actually on the range, whereas some people will make it into their profile picture on social media. I am however much more interested in movies and the making of them. A large majority of my YouTube library and watchlist has been essays on why this movie sucks or what made that film great. I think a lot of that stems from renting movies in high school from the school library. I'd watch the VHS tapes at night at low volume so my parents wouldn't hear (I wasn't actually allowed to watch movies on my TV/VCR unit, but that is a story for later) and become captivated with what made movies good, explicitly Casablanca *(1942) and its night at the Oscars.*

GRINDR

Pranks at the office are as old as the cliche itself. They build comradery, increase morale, and shorten the days until you can go home again. They do these things for everyone except the mark of the prank. In this case that was me, and it was a stain that I have to wear with me to this day.

For most of my adult life I had been the target of a confused sexual being. Was it because I was sexually assaulted when I was seven years old? I doubt it, and apart from my family, I have only told two people in my life what happened, and the details shared were vague, believe that. I never followed up by asking my mother about questions I may have had, and I never told anyone in the military that it happened.

Then there was the sexually charged Cal Rastall in his dorm room at UW-Green Bay, the definition of desperate. One night, before being catfished was a common term in the lexicon of a naive, tunnel-visioned young man such as myself, I was led to believe that someone wanted to come to my dorm room one night for relations. This was all done via AOL Instant Messenger, and no one on the swim team who I was debating my decision with, who lived in the same building as me, thought this was a good idea. Unfortunately for me, I didn't care, and the person was invited, only to realize it was not actually a woman, but a man from my Intro to Public Administration course. Because I'm the bigger man, I will not mention their name, but since that day I have worn the stench of the swimmer who made out with that guy. It made coming back to Green Bay or keeping in contact with old teammates a bit awkward.

Finally, we have the deployment Grindr story. Someone made a profile of me. A Whiskey member (who has requested Personal Identifiable Information be redacted from this book), who is gay, showed me the profile as proof. He came to my room because he was concerned and confused and wanted to know the truth from the horse's mouth. For that, I tip my hat to him. At first, I thought it was funny, almost honored to be the butt of a joke. I mean, if someone is going that far out of their way to bust your balls, you must be making some sort of impact. I laughed at the photo, explained it was not me, and asked for the profile to be marked as spam or something that flagged it as an untrue profile.

That story garnered some laughs on my way to the chow hall the next morning because it was that surreal, but I didn't think much more about it until the profile came back and started speaking on my behalf. If there is one thing in this world I hate, it's someone speaking on my behalf when I'm more than capable of doing it myself. When the person on the other end said that I was secretly in the closet and my wife and children are all a show, I went from a place of hehe-haha deployment humor to not laughing at all. What made it worse was the distance locator said the correspondent was 0.1 miles away. Because I hadn't talked to anyone else outside of the unit, it was coming from within the unit.

This was something I could not shake for the rest of my time on the deployment as we'll read later. Even my best friend on the deployment confronted me to ask if I was gay. It has been a series of unfortunate events in this arena, but it's also part of life. I'm not minimizing what has happened to me, but I'm aware enough to know that no one has a perfect life no matter the projection they display for the rest of the world to see.

16 Mar 2020
Day 28

Happy "Stone Cold" Steve Austin Day. That's right, Austin 3:16 is alive and well. For a day that had me doing almost nothing, I think there is plenty to say.

We started the self-imposed quarantine from Fort Bliss and consequently Freedom Crossing. No more Chipotle, Buffalo Wild Wings, or Texas Roadhouse. Dairy Queen and the movie theater, too, are gone. Everyone is losing their minds on this coronavirus. Captain Kahler recommended a book on Audible about crowd hysteria. Now I must choke down these last hours of *Grant*. Still not finished.

I also finished *Parasite* (2019). It is a good thing, one thinks, to find myself researching afterward on YouTube the movies that are worth the time. For example, I only looked on IMDB.com for another movie I watched, Seth Rogan and Charlize Theron's *Long Shot* (2019). It was cute.

There was no class today. My first day off since coming here. I laid in bed and either YouTubed or napped. I'm much more awake than I should be, and I did not exercise when I had every opportunity to. Didn't eat breakfast; large lunch, but MRE for dinner. Did you know one MRE is only 1,250 calories?

Chief ended up talking to the enlisted crew. Hopefully that's the end of it.

Postscript: This was the beginning of the end of good times. The real fun of living in a world with coronavirus began on this day in my life. Up until then we didn't need masks, it was optional, but the levees broke after this day. MREs, or Meals Ready to Eat, weren't bad in onesies or twosies, but when it was your main course for days, it added to the grind. One of the few fortunate things about my time in Texas was there was internet available in my room, and the Wi-Fi was strong enough to continue everyday life.

19 Mar 2020
Day 29, 30 & 31

Oh boy, another three-page entry, and wouldn't you know it's laundry day. I think there is a lot to unpack here so let's take it away, shall we?

Our flight to Qatar has been cancelled. We were supposed to leave in two days, but the coronavirus hysteria is in full bloom. All professional sports are either suspended or cancelled for the remainder of the seasons.

Someone I know made a racist joke that one guy in China sneezes and he lost 20% of his 401k. I'm moderately anxious about my own Thrift Savings Plan, or TSP, but at least I'm buying stocks when they are low. It will eventually have to bounce back, but this might just be my 2008.

Aaron Eastman is losing his mind calling this "his war." Good for him to get into the fight. Sounds like Saori will not be throwing Josiah a birthday party this year, and the sakura (cherry blossom tree) will not be as celebrated as in years past.

I honestly don't know what to think of COVID. My opinion is obviously skewed, because I have been living in Japan and been cooped up in relative isolation since coming back to America. Like I told Dylan, no one minds public health until it directly affects them.

Past couple of days I have been on a shopping spree of sorts. Mostly I'm buying patches and Wisconsin and Japan flags of different colors and designs. I was yesterday-years old when I learned the generic name for Velcro is hook'n'loop. Blew my mind.

I also paid for Atticus' doctor bill that occurred in October 2019 for his skin. It was urgent care and $376. My ignorant mind thought Tricare would just take care of it. Nope! And now I'm in America with limited access to everything. I'll work through it.

Finally, I might just purchase another pair of shoes for gym purposes. I'm on the fence, but I might.

For good news today, we are complete with our Army training as of today. The rest of our time will be waiting. I truly hope I can light the necessary fire under myself and continue making personal improvements. For the last week or so I have been delinquent on going to the gym and relying on the fasting to hold me over. Admittedly, and without access to a scale that is reliable, I do seem to be shrinking. It helps that I don't snack when I'm not eating a meal.

Oh, literally 75 minutes before being told that we weren't flying out on time, I dropped 30 lb of things enroute to Japan and 31 lb of gear forwarded to Kandahar Airfield (KAF). Altogether, that was $154. Amazing; certainly did not look forward to telling Saori about that one.

I finally got to place theory to test. I thought and wrote about how I needed to work on my follower skills. Our PAO is killing me. I lay out a plan, she overrules it. I give an idea and she runs with it like it's hers. Either our styles are very similar or very far apart. Luckily, I have a couple of the First Classes working with me on getting over this mental hurdle I keep finding myself bumping into. Anyway, a lot of that drama aside, I've been asked to draft our first article. No idea on the word count yet. Tomorrow we will supposedly have breakfast as a PAO team.

Over the next couple of days, I hope to clean my gun for the first time. Also, I would like to rearrange my room for me to not sleep in the bottom bunk, but with no bunk at all. There is always room for less YouTube, and hopefully with more light in the bunk I will be encouraged to read more. I'm just really bummed that so much stuff was packed so prematurely. Really needed that Tylenol today.

Postscript: I absolutely loved writing entries while doing laundry. There was something quiet about the laundromat, and, less poetically, there was a table to write on. You might say that I was constantly looking for that big idea. Although I didn't know what it was, my mind was constantly searching for a project I could sink my teeth into. Yes, I cleaned my weapon only when I absolutely needed to, unlike some folks in our unit who did it routinely after each use. I was convinced that if I needed to use it, I was probably going to die anyway. The PAO drama was something that entertained me more than anything. We all have problems, and this is what I hung my hat on. I wish I could have fought world hunger instead of focusing on something so silly, but that was the time I lived in.

20 Mar 2020
Day 32

What a day, yet what all happened? We technically only had a training meeting at 0900 and evening muster. No fear because that was all we officially had on the books.

I thought my training meeting went a little sideways, but it was progressive overall. Ended up jotting down three pages of notes afterward. Who knows if anyone except me will look at it now or later.

I was going to have a PAO meeting at 1300, but it was postponed until tomorrow. Will most certainly write notes in preparation for it after this post.

Something I meant to include in yesterday's post was that it was on the 30-day mark when I first felt the first pangs of being homesick. I don't know if I should be telling Saori about it. Watching the boys on video chat, I can see them becoming unglued and it's only been a month. How Chelsea Wydra did it, or how any forward-deployed spouse who time after time raises their family in the continued absence of the Sailor is beyond me.

I reported a gas leak tonight and the fire department had to evacuate the building. Continued working on the command coin with HN Valdez. It's shaping up and we're expecting the first proof soon. No gym today.

Postscript: I no longer have those meeting minutes, and I'm a shameful historian because of it.

ME AND THE CAP'N MAKING IT HAPPEN

There are some people who cross your life's path who you just seem to gravitate towards. Captain Daniel Kahler, MC, USNR, was one of those fellows that I'll remember for a long time. My encounters with him are sprinkled throughout this book, and he's one of those people I wish I could spend much more time focusing on because I just found him that interesting.

Some of the best stories are forged from the humblest of beginnings. When we were all packed into that room in Norfolk, we barely knew one another. There was a divide between the officers and enlisted, and an even wider gap between active duty and reservists. On the Whiskey Rotation there were no enlisted reservists, but on that day in Norfolk I did not know that. All our eyes were peeled like we were looking for stray bullets, but we were looking at everyone's rank instead. Rank is our cue for how to address someone and whether we can let out any unsavory four-letter words in their presence. It's our chance to build immediate bridges when we're all stranded on an island of isolation although we all sat in a crowded room.

In comes this Captain, a "full bird," as we say when addressing an O-6. In the other branches we call them Colonels, but here in the Navy it's Captain. He had the thickest glasses of anyone on the team and this giant Michigan State University class ring on (I later found out it was from 1989). He was bebopping around with an executive presence, which was mildly intimidating at first, but that was how I met Captain Kahler.

Possibly my second memory of him was when he asked me about my last name. Because I loved the story, I told him when I was about 19 years old, I worked at a Ponderosa Steakhouse on the eastside of Green Bay, WI, and there was a retired linguistics teacher from the university down the road who would eat there from time to time. On one fateful day I was his server and he looked at my nametag and dissected it with "ras" meaning river and "tal" meaning mountain, so my name was Swiss-German for "river in the mountain." Not knowing anything about the good Captain, he was like, "I know a little German, and that doesn't mean river." To this day I haven't looked it up to see who was right or wrong, and I prefer to keep the integrity of the memory instead of knowing the facts.

When we were in Texas, of course the longest-serving officer had his own room, right? Well, not in Whiskey. By the time we left, not even the Commanding Officer had her own room. It was just the Executive Officer and me (although I lived in the toilet paper supply closet). Captain Kahler bunked with the Chief of Surgery, Commander John Mayberry. Two old guys who every time I walked past their room were probably listening to jazz and reading something. The bathrooms were communal, and we'd run into one another while shaving. Without hesitation, and as a term of endearment I'd always say the same thing, "Hey Cap'n! What's Hap'n?" Hopefully Post Cereal doesn't read this and demand a royalty check, nor should they since Cap'n Crunch was technically a commander.

Captain Kahler was the last person I talked to before we parted ways as a rotation at the Baltimore Airport when we came home, and I don't think it could have ended any better for me. I think of him often and still repeat some of the gems that he was kind enough to share with me when we were together.

22 Mar 2020
Day 33 & 34

I wish all days were like today. Woke up early, got to the gym (and did remarkably well, which I'll get to), came back, had a cup of coffee, sat and read the *Reader's Digest* my mom sent me, shared a few "good mornings" with folks in the building, spoke with Rich on Skype, and this was all done before cleaning stations at 0830. Oh, and I called Saori mid-gym.

As I write, it's only 0901 on the 22nd, but I have enough to say to get me two pages. The room reconfiguration is paying dividends. It even caught the attention and ire of a few First Classes. It's clean, bright, and fitting to the way I want it for my comfort. That's one thing of many that Greg Fall taught me. How I wish I was still working with him.

This safety/supply/facilities gig is starting to really either be more important or they are starting to notice. It feels good in any case. Which brings us neatly along to our PAO meeting yesterday. I thought there was tension, and there very well could have been. The direction bothers me or at least the presentation of order. It sounds like I have the corner on the newsletter, *The Whiskey Ration.* Except I don't. LCDR Fitzgerald is very possessive of her product, and I can respect that to a point. I would like to see more delegation and trust, but I believe this will come with time and proof of value to the team. Either way, I am finding myself very busy writing articles, which is right where I want to be.

It just occurred to me that I hold writing so close to me because it is one medium that will live on long after I'm gone. Still on the fence about if I want to transcribe these words onto a computer document. Who knows, maybe my time in Kandahar will be extra special and publication worthy.

As mentioned before, I was at the gym today. I was inspired by Jocko Willinik's Ted Talk of his book *Extreme Ownership.* That dude is so intimidating and intense. Did the trick though because there I was pounding pavement. Well, treadmill pavement. Last time I ran seriously was March 6. Wow, I could only do 17:30 at a 4.5 mph pace. I don't know why, but I completed the 30:00 jog at a 4.5 pace. Looks like I get to fail upwards tomorrow starting at 5.0. I also did some free weights. Bench 135 lb, 3 sets of 8 reps. Then went to incline. One set of 115 lb of six reps. My arms were already fried. Then did a basic plank set.

Postscript: I'm not sure why that free weight set was so memorable to me, but it was. Possibly because of how much my body hurt afterward. It would make sense to keep it up, but consistency on this deployment was never my thing no matter how much I tried or wrote about it. Even in my frustration of learning about myself, I always tried to remain objective. It didn't always work, but working through my thoughts with LCDR Fitzgerald definitely gave me something to do.

23 Mar 2020
Day 35

I've been feeling like a dog chasing cars today. So many options and possibilities running through my mind I wouldn't know what to do if I caught one and sunk my teeth into it.

For example, I was on the treadmill (more on that in a moment) and the idea of writing an *Opie & The Foreman* memoir of how I built and sustained the Sconnie Sailor Moving Company passed through my mind. That's not the only thing on my mind, I want to stand up the Whiskey Rotation Facebook page. I want to read good books, have meaningful conversations, and make an impact. Yes, I'm making an impact on my children's lives, but that's not what I mean.

Told my friend Aaron Eastman the "military perspective" on how some people are going to die and it will seem so preventable, etc. What I really said worth noting was the longer I'm in America the more I'm reminded and see Americans' gross sense of entitlement. It really is sickening to see on a micro level, although on a macro scale it made us, Americans, what we are now.

Treadmill left more to be desired, sort of. Started out as promised at 5.0 mph and kept it there for 1 mile, or 12:00 before having to use the restroom. Came back and did another walk/jog at 5.0/3.0 for 30 minutes. Overall time was 42 minutes and 3 miles.

Postscript: I'm not sure what I thought about this deployment and what would happen. Someone close to me said that the number one enemy I would face was boredom. I suppose I internalized that as having literally nothing to do, and I began to plot my time out with things I wanted to do. As we would see, boredom was not my enemy, and I was nowhere near completing a fraction of the jobs I wanted to get done. Some projects are still on the backburner, but I really did think I would be having hours to myself to create worlds within my mind.

26 Mar 2020
Day 36, 37 & 38

I wasn't supposed to take this long before writing, but now I suddenly have something to say. First, I've been watching a lot of movies. Yesterday I watched *JoJo Rabbit* (2019), and I really liked it. Before watching it, I wondered how they could pull off Nazis being funny. They did though, but it's also not that hard to imagine when the director of *Thor: Ragnarök* (2017) is at the helm.

I also watched the WWE Studio film *Fighting with my Family*. Because I don't like Paige the wrestler to begin with, I blame this for taking so long to see it. Plus, it's a WWE Studio film; it's not how good it is, but how bad it is. Honestly, it was charming, but I'm always weird about biopics.

Last I watched *Midway*. I found it a film more suited to the active duty/veteran's ilk. There were many parts where I think filmmakers captured the military and "got it," but the editing was awful. Talk about getting tossed around from one incoherent scene to the next.

Next up we had a suspected case of coronavirus within the ranks. We were pretty much house arrested to our rooms and hallways. This should explain all the movies. As it turns out it was a negative test, and restrictions were lifted that afternoon. With that said, still no fly-out date, but I have requested Saori mail everything to KAF instead of here. I have the Internet and enough books to keep me entertained.

Speaking of, I finished the book LT Scott Byrd shared, *Elephant in the Room* by Tommy Tomlinson. It was a quick read, and there were parts I definitely connected with and enjoyed sharing with LT. We find ourselves sharing a lot of "isms" with one another. He has challenged me to memorize Kipling's *If,* and I believe I'm up for the challenge.

I was having huge pangs to start my memoir about the Sconnie Sailor Moving Company. If I had my laptop, it would have been started. Maybe I can use this time to draw an outline to properly organize my thoughts because I think that's the part that is holding me back, getting stuck in the middle and creating bulk. Within my mind's eye I can see the opening/start with many of my projects, but it gets hazy in the middle. I don't think many authors believe their work is anything special. I mean, did Harper Lee finish *To Kill a Mockingbird* and think it was going to be an American literature masterpiece, or was she just happy it was published? It's interesting where some roads take us.

Which leads me to my final page and thoughts. It may be my final mystery, but I don't know why I'm so attractive to gay men. From Jason to Dan to tonight. A nurse corps Lieutenant was caressing my thigh beneath the table tonight. First, I said, "No," and he stopped. Then he started again, and I had to firmly say, "Lieutenant." He stopped, and I traded out my cards to go report what had happened. To HM1 Wilson, again. Chief Atangan is like, "Whatever you want to do." Unfortunately, punching him in the face is not a viable option. Chief obviously told Senior, and that's when the interviews happened. Everyone at the spades table that night was taken aside. Who knows what will happen, but we aren't even in Afghanistan yet, and this is getting old. It's not much fun when you're the target.

On that note, playing spades with officers is like drinking Fireball. Maybe it sounds like a fun idea, but it doesn't take long to learn it's probably the worst decision you're going to make in quite some time. It was interesting watching the XO play Cards Against Humanity with only enlisted.

Tomorrow is a CO call and I think I'm going to touch on good order and discipline.

Postscript: These are the posts that caused me to think twice before sharing in my story. For some reason I still think it's necessary to redact the accuseds' names and keep their dignity intact by penning anonymity next to their actions. What I mean by this is, people I know and who love me will read some of these pages and get a new clear understanding of what I meant when I said my deployment wasn't much fun. Sure, there were plenty of other reasons, COVID-19 being among those, but I decided to share this story because to me it was special, and I wanted others who will never get the same opportunities I did to somehow experience what I had to. As it turns out, the officer in question was hauled into the stateroom of the XO with the company of the Chiefs present. Although I was left alone, it didn't take away some awkward moments for the next six months. No, I did not talk about good order and discipline, I was just in a mood when I wrote that. As it turns out, the XO bonding with the enlisted was one of the best parts of the whole experience. Made him human.

30 Mar 2020
Day 39, 40, 41 & 42

Wouldn't you know, another laundry day. LCDR Tom Warner was kind enough to buy new pens and sunscreen for me, and that is what I'm writing with now. Of course, I paid him back. Not sure how it was only $7, but I'm not going to complain.

These pens are 0.5's. I have come to prefer 0.7's the most, but at least I can go about my days free from fear about running out of ink.

For the past couple of days, I was watching the #1 show on Netflix called *Tiger King*. That show is wild, I doubt anyone could have thought up such a bizarre story. It was a rare binge, but worth it. Also playing a lot of spades. Right now, I'm in a losing stretch, and I think it is really getting my mood down.

Actually, there are a number of things that are bringing down my mood, and I hope to examine more later within these pages. I don't know why, but I am daydreaming a lot more about cooking and baking when I get back. It seems like something cool to do with the boys, especially the baking.

Today facilities turned on the air-conditioning and blew out the dust and sand in the vents. It promptly fell all over my room and onto everything. Half my laundry is dusty/sandy sheets. Yesterday country singer Joe Diffie died from coronavirus. He was 61. Kenny Rogers is also dead. Being in Fort Bliss is not a very lucky place for good news, but to be fair he was like 80.

Days have been very slow and uneventful. I wish I could share what exactly goes on in a day, but for the most part it is just blah. I look back, and I have more to say about what hasn't happened rather than what did. Even more to the point, I'm most mentally torn up about what should have been done.

This gig as the supply/facilities Petty Officer is getting to me. Am I not managing my expectations appropriately? There are just so many entitled people who just take what isn't theirs without asking. In my mind I took a serious misstep when I used Chief AT's position and influence to try and get a car bench seat that was just taken from the storage closet. Turns out an O-4, Lieutenant Commander, unilaterally thought the seat would look dandy in their room. I was just frustrated, and it read so in my group message. More importantly, Chief did not appreciate it and my shame is what hurts the most.

My articles for *The Whiskey Ration* Issue #1 are complete. They are okay; not my best work, but there was close to seven pages of content. I foresee LCDR Fitzgerald somehow pissing some or all of us off in one way or another. Today she upset HN Valdez by essentially stealing a project from her. Valdez went on and on about Fitzgerald and how she treats other people on the PAO staff. Her alpha persona is going to stunt her free help and labor. I hope to never treat or be perceived how she is.

My diet has gone to hell. Hopefully today is the first day I can get back on track with the intermittent fasting. Missed breakfast and held out until 1430 for a peanut butter and jelly sandwich. Just one, too.

From what I'm told, the "windy" months around here are March, April, and May. So far, the reports from the locals are correct. On top of that, it gets windier the later in the day we go. This means I'm in no mood to go to the track. What I ought to do is just wake up earlier. Because I didn't nap today, this might just happen.

Finally, the last thing I will be talking about is *Opie & The Foreman.* I wrote my first page today. Surprisingly it went smoother than I deserved. What I wasn't expecting was how often I veered from my outline. I must assume this is good and bad. Good because I clearly have something to say, and I'm getting enough content to make the paper bleed, but bad because this will force me into my least favorite part of writing: editing and revising. As Johnny Depp is famous for never watching his own movies, I absolutely hate reading my own work. Come to it, I don't care much for hearing my own voice either. Maybe that is yet another reason why I prefer to write. I like the internal voice more than what my ears hear.

Oh, I officially applied for graduation. That cost $306. I checked on Thomas Edison State University graduate programs too, and they were not cheap, like $24K without tuition assistance. Maybe I'll look at UW-Madison programs too... (long sigh).

Postscript: There is a lot of good material within this post. Not sure why, but Joe Diffie's death really got to me and helped me believe that this coronavirus was real. One of the best purchases I made, though, was his greatest hits album. His song "Home" still gives me goosebumps, but then again, many songs about home do. I used Lieutenant Commander Warner's gift until the day I returned to Japan. In my group message regarding the van bench, I said that "Chief AT wants it back." Chief promptly replied to everyone that he in fact did not say that. Because that chair was in a room I was designated guardian over, and it went missing, I took it upon myself to get it back with whatever means I needed to. There is a right way and a wrong way of doing things, and I found out the latter that day.

1 April 2020
Day 43 & 44

Happy birthday to all the Chief Petty Officers out there, past and present. We are still in McGregor with no end in sight. From what the Commanding Officer (otherwise written as "CO" or "Skipper") was trying to convey yesterday, the Exception to Policy request for medical units to travel during this travel ban has been denied. There is a lot of limbo and it's starting to get to us all, myself included.

It's not even 0900 and I'm journaling so it might serve as a therapeutic tool. I know I'm getting amped up about the armory/supply closet/food pantry/random conference room. I guess it is my job to clean it, but I think I'm going to tell Chief that I'm not going to clean it if people are still going in there getting food during cleaning stations. It's not time for second breakfast, or even their first. They know when breakfast is, and it's not during cleaning stations! It is really upsetting me.

On one hand, why should I even care? Maybe it's because I don't want to live in a lawless land. Possibly this an ownership issue. Am I not being assertive enough? What is my land? The last thing I want to be is a pawn and quickly dismissed. I want my job to have credibility and be taken seriously. We'll talk to the First Classes first and see where their minds are at.

Last night I had a good conversation with Captain Kahler, my "doppelganger," and LCDR John Stewart. It was a mini course on promotion and career planning. Captain said something interesting as a recommendation how I might be better off if I cast my line out a little further in regard to not limiting myself. Maybe it was just the wording that piqued my interest. Because I'm writing about it now should imply how much I appreciate the talk, and hopefully there is more.

This morning I had my random chest pain. It's hard to describe; it's the second time it has happened. Not radiating pain, elephant-on-chest feeling or jaw pain. A centralized acute pain. Possibly anxiety, but I was sitting in a chair looking at Instagram. Nothing at the forefront of my mind about what I was thinking "I am anxious about THIS." Possibly my sub-consciousness talking to me? I'm fine now, it lasted only five minutes, maybe.

Knocked out a couple of pages for *Opie & The Foreman: An American's Chase of the Dream.* I'm very thankful I ended up drafting that outline after all. Good to read a lot today and think.

Postscript: When someone is bored, it is amazing the lengths they will go to in order to feel entertained. This is seen in many ways, and the way I did this was by wanting to be the man in the high castle of the toilet paper closet. Looking back on it, I can't help but feel shame. On the other hand, I was so focused on being "the man" on the deployment that I wasn't going to let some people who I felt were making bad decisions cause a blemish on my reputation for being dependable. Little could I see at the time, it was my reaction that caused the blemish, if at all. Just because you're feeling, seeing, or experiencing something does not mean that it's actually reality.

2 April 2020
Day 45

Believe it or not, I am on duty right now. I've taken other watches, but this is my first watch that I was assigned to in a long time. I wonder if this is how often I would be standing watch at a "real" command.

Pretty lazy day with only a pinch of drama. Apparently, the triad spoke with Victor Rotation. This morning at muster the CO and XO get up to their jaw-jacking, and afterwards Senior Chief essentially dismantles everything that was said. I think we caught a glimpse of frustration. There are like five plans still in play ranging from we stay at McGregor until we fly out, to getting pimped out to other missions (there are plenty going on right now), to even sending us home for good. In one dream I had, I acted essentially as WALL-E where everyone took leave to go back home until 14 days before we fly out, but I just stayed here, alone.

Made what I thought was progress last night; I finished the first draft of my introduction chapter of *Opie & The Foreman.* It was Google-shared with Dr. Christina "Dearest" Solomon just to see if I'm on the right track.

So, I'm getting lonely for Japanese, well, everything. I have increased my YouTube for Japan stuff and watching Netflix content. Now I'm watching *My Husband Doesn't Fit.* #Nippon

Postscript: The officer and enlisted communities are different. They must be. To grossly simplify the contrast between the two, officers are focused on mission, and enlisted are about the people. Sometimes at recognition boards such as Sailor of the Year, the question will be asked, "What is more important, the mission or the Sailor?" It really is a "chicken or the egg" question, and some people feel like they should take a side. It's my belief that both are critical and to believe one is more important than the other is neither capable nor worthy of a leadership post in the Navy. To that end, there are obvious reasons why officers are written about while "it's not the Chief way" for the senior enlisted to receive as much credit as they deserve. When Senior took us, the enlisted, aside, he no doubt had a horseshoe of chewing tobacco and illustrated the situation in terms we could understand, usually punctuated with four-letter words. Our worlds are different, and they should be; we have different missions to focus on.

3 April 2020
Day 46

Today was quasi-chill yet teeming with potential. The mornings just escape from me. For the past couple of days, I have been waking up at 0730. Then I get my head about me for the 0800 muster where I have to be out in formation by 0750. That generally gives me enough time to turn my Wi-Fi back on to check important messages and Line app communication from home. It's too late by then to call the boys, but once a day when they are up is so far working out.

Then it's straight to cleaning stations where I take my job cleaning the armory possibly more serious than it needs to be. After that I sent a couple of messages and walked to Mayor Cell to submit a couple trouble tickets. I get a kick talking to the facilities guys. I tell them that Mayor Cell is my Olive Garden because when I'm there, I'm family.

Since I got back though, I've just been chilling. As long as I stay away from YouTube, I think I'm going to be okay. I am awaiting light switch maintenance for my room though. Requested stamps and envelopes from the local shoppette. Hope it works out. I'm about to officially redraft my outline. Hopefully Christina will write back.

Day 14 of "self-quarantine."

Postscript: This was my first experience on an Army base. Fort Bliss in Texas is huge, and it's in the middle of nowhere. Where we were, the McGregor Range, was even farther into the middle of nowhere. There were terms I had to quickly learn. For example, the Galley is where I get food, but now it's called the DFAC. To this day I don't know what Mayor Cell is except that it was like the headquarters building where facilities staff were sitting around waiting for the next problem to land on their desk. They were a good group of guys who took the time to help me out. I came in there with my hands at my side, palms open with admission that the people I represented were giving them first world problems to fix, but it was my job to make sure it got done. They played ball with me and I'm thankful for them.

Dr. Christina "Dearest" Solomon

People come and go out of your lives with only a few precious ones that you can hold onto. My friendship with Christina Solomon is one of those folks, and my story with her is woven so tightly it warrants some backstory and context. She is littered throughout this text and for good reason, she helped me remain sane when few could.

I didn't always hail from Baraboo, Wisconsin. Although born in Appleton, Wisconsin, my parents took my brother and me to a small town outside of Nashville, Tennessee, called Hendersonville from fifth grade to sixth grade. These are forgettable years that are easily brushed over when thinking about my life, but the only upside was in 1999 when we welcomed my last sibling, Maxwell, to the family. From the start of seventh grade, I called Baraboo my hometown, and I still do.

Christina Solomon was always a friend, but usually the friend of the girls who I was crushing on at the time. We were in band class together, ran in the same circles, and always knew one another, but were never close. One day I was whining about my poor dating record with one of her friends, and she finally had enough of me when she snapped and placed me in a headlock trying to get me to snap out of my melancholy state. She was fair and dainty and the exact opposite of me in many regards. She called me "Freak" and I responded with calling her "Dearest." She has since stopped wanting to openly use her moniker, but to this day she will always be Dearest to me.

After graduation from high school, we went our separate paths. I struggled to keep school a serious priority and she excelled in academia. With the help of Mark Zuckerberg, we kept loose tabs on one another until I joined the Navy. She had taken a year to study and teach in Korea while I was in Japan, and, being lonely, I began to conjure up wild ideas about the possibility of an "us." It was short-lived, and I remained attracted to her mind, thoughts, and friendship. Whenever I would travel home on leave, she would be home in Baraboo, usually in the summers, and we could talk for hours over tea or simply at my parent's dining room table.

Dearest went on to earn her doctorate degree and took up the name Dr. Dearest. I am extremely proud of her and what she has accomplished, and she has been polite to commend me on what I have done. After I met Saori and grew into my marriage, it became different between Dearest and I. It had to, but the friendship always remained.

When I was in Texas, we began a journey of building off on that friendship. It was platonic and it still is. In the most asexual way, I can describe I will forever remain fond of my friend. We can debate and argue, laugh and cry together. We do not dwell on the past of high school, but do not stop to work through some of the problems we faced during those times. We talk of a future and what it means to find our paths and relationships.

We want different things in life, and that is great. It doesn't dismiss the fact though that we both find solitude in each other's company, and it is a relationship I will cherish for as long as I remain a part of her life. Dr. Dearest remains one of the good ones, and it was during this deployment that we unapologetically used one another to work through some tough times that I will always remember.

4 April 2020
Day 47

Don't look now, but I think I'm starting to find my groove. This is what, the third consecutive day I'm inputting a journal entry?

The days of monotony have some benefits. For one, it makes planning my day that much easier. Although last night I hope I decided on something I can stick to. There I was, going on a walk, and I was thinking about my future. I need to get back to a calorie restricted diet and increase my output of physical activity. My 3.5 mile walk yesterday left my legs a little sore this morning. To me, that's a problem. Walking should not do this. Back to just water and coffee, and only one meat at dinner. Nor more second helpings. A walk in the morning after cleaning and one more in the evening where I might put in a little more effort while it's cooler.

Had another good night with the book. Luckily, I am free to write and write and write because there is no word count. One concern that did pop up was the flow, structure, and placement of paragraphs and stories. I felt I went on too many tangents. I want to say everything, but does it fit and flow for the reader? Right now, I need to concentrate on just getting words on the pages. Today is Saturday, and it's laundry day. Spirits are up and I'm being productive.

Postscript: One of the biggest drawbacks to the toilet paper closet was I did not have a desk, or my own computer. There is something to be said about writing comfortably. What ended up happening was a lot of writing that was done in my mind, and I would try to recreate it on a notepad for when Lieutenant Byrd was able to spare his laptop. I really like, however, that I was thinking critically about my problems at hand. There is something to be said for typing something beyond an assigned paper for college and really exploring creative writing.

5 April 2020
Day 48

I wonder if this is how prisoners feel when trying to pass the time. Are they able to spend the days in their bed if they choose? It's only 1300 and I feel like a solid day has already come to pass. I have read, napped, Netflixed, YouTubed, and Facebook Messaged some friends.

There are no consequences, just hang out and let your imagination run wild. I like it, except that I wish I had my own computer. Each evening I borrow LT Scott Byrd's after dinner. At night, after my walk, I will spend a couple hours on the book. What I'm trying to do is use the day to brainstorm and collect my thoughts. So far it is an agreeable schedule. I really like how I can just read and write. My problem is as I am writing, and just how into the bushes do I want to get? There needs to be a balance between tone, style, and I suppose ultimate intent. My goal is to make this 250 pages. Until then, I need to just get the words on the page.

Last night I started adding squats into my laps. At each corner of the track, I would do 10, and I did that for 3 laps, so 120 air squats. Not only did I feel them at the time (I felt powerful), but this morning I was a bit stiff, and that was the goal. Not shredded, but sore.

Postscript: Writing is a beautiful thing. There is structure, but it's free. There are rules, but you are the boss. For the longest time I thought that Harper Lee wrote To Kill a Mockingbird *in essentially one take on the typewriter. Like she had one chance and it became an American classic. I now have firsthand experience that the likelihood of that happening was very low. Repeatedly taking notes and letting the words settle like fine sediment is a process. Should anyone take an interest in becoming an author, and asked me for advice, I would place having patience ahead of talent if you want to reach success.*

7 April 2020
Day 49 & 50

Happy birthday Josiah Oki Michael Rastall. You are five years old today, and I know this is affecting your mother a lot more than me. By now I've come to realize that birthdays divisible by 5 are a bigger deal than others, but any birthday to a child is a big deal. No matter which way you cut it, I am not there to share the day with you. Moreover, your birthday is the first of my three sons' birthdays.

This is uncharted territory for me as a Navy man. Some guys go into a career by doing this, being absent. Where it doesn't strike me as weird the divorce rate is so high, it does make me think how some people can be so married to the sea. Like Willem Dafoe in *Spider Man* (2002). Just kidding, in the *Lighthouse* (2019). Clearly my mind was in other places. Yesterday I got a care package from Baraboo. Inside was a *Reader's Digest*, beef jerky links, "Easter" trail mix, and a book about the olympians of Wisconsin. I did not know there were so many of them.

Yesterday was a bad day for me because I let my feelings get to me. Apparently, there was a four-star general who came to McGregor Range on a helicopter. Sadly, I didn't catch the name, but my first thought is who would actually want to come here? What really started to cook my grits was how much it seemingly spooked the Skipper. Our classes were canceled, I wasn't allowed to wear Navy clothes, and pretty much out of sight, out of mind, was the guidance. It bothers me that hiding was the plan of action rather than at least doing nothing to change the course of action. If we are wrong, we'd be corrected; if we were asked, we had immediate access to the highest levels of military leadership.

Instead, I stayed in my room for 90% of my day and watched three movies: *Zombieland 2: Double Tap* (2019), *Drunk Parents* (2019), and *The Lincoln Lawyer* (2011). *Double Tap* was charming and aligned with its predecessor. *Lincoln Lawyer* was great because I like lawyer movies, but *Drunk Parents* was absolute trash.

Today I asked Senior Chief if he'd think less of me if I left the PAO team. He said he wouldn't. I'm not sure what to do, but luckily I have his blessing. The first issue is not even published. I'm looking for my out. Didn't do any writing last night. LT Byrd needed the computer, so I stayed happy knowing I completed my first chapter after the introduction. I also did not go for a walk because I was so sore. I've added body weight squats and delayed muscle soreness to boot. I'm going to call Dr. "Dearest" Solomon today. Jazzed.

Postscript: Whenever I speculate on the actions of the highest levels of Whiskey Rotation leadership, it's important to remind everyone that is exactly what it was, speculation. Who knows what the absolute truth was, but at the time, in the moment, that was my truth. It also showcased me being bored and looking for conflict. Missing big milestones like Josiah's birthday, and later my child's birth, could be viewed in a couple of ways. I decided not to take the "woe is me" mentality but think of it as a badge of honor. That is what being deployed is about, having to miss some things in the short run while serving a higher purpose. The shift in how you view a problem can really turn a situation on its head, and it helped me cope.

9 April 2020
Day 51 & 52

What a time to be alive. Yesterday I may have heard the most Navy thing ever. We finally have progress, but it aligns firmly with Navy logic. Of Whiskey Rotation, as of now, only the reservist component is being booked to travel to Afghanistan. The active-duty personnel remain in a holding pattern with our futures undetermined. There is absolutely zero word on the outlook for me.

This of course leads the rumor mill to lose its damn mind. Are we being sent to our parent commands to be summoned later? Will we be authorized to take leave? Will the whole thing just be cancelled? No one who matters knows. Senior Chief Wink is super transparent, but I don't know if that is the right play. Being open with facts and official word is great, but once personal opinions are involved, I hope it doesn't become haunting later on.

Last night I got on the *New Pope* train. It's the follow-up season to Jude Law's *Young Pope* on HBO. John Malkovich is the lead, and after two episodes I really like it. For some reason I napped a lot yesterday, more so than normal. Today I seemed to have sustained enough energy despite only getting 5.5 hours of sleep.

My morning today has been productive enough. Cleaned out the armory/food pantry, read much of the *Reader's Digest* Mom sent with a thermos of coffee by my side. Then I did a load of laundry. Afterwards I plan to get some laps in, take a nap, and prepare for dinner.

Oh, yesterday I won an auction on eBay for a Chromebook. New ones on Amazon were like $300, much more expensive than I remember. Including shipping and tax, I paid $125 for mine. Bought a mouse and batteries off Amazon too. Until these items arrive, I think I will suspend *Opie & The Foreman.*

There is a growing sense of guilt within my marrow, and with LT Byrd supposedly leaving with the rest of the reservists, I'm not going to have a choice either way. Maybe today I'll shop for soap, stamps, and envelopes.

The First Classes, who risked their lives on a PX run, forgot the single bar of soap I requested, but certainly didn't forget their tobacco. Holy cow, I'm beginning to sound like a righteous "former tobacco user." That's gross.

I'm not bored, just excited for the rest of my life to start. I'm all about daydreaming of the things I want to do once I get back to Japan.

Postscript: This day was a big shift in the tempo of life in Texas. We knew something was happening in the nebulous, and each day was an exciting time to be alive. As busy as I was in the toilet paper closet, it pales in comparison to the post office clerks who retrieved the mail for Whiskey Rotation. Think about it, I was buying soap, stamps, and envelopes online, and I'm just one person. We were not able to shop anywhere, and that was a very snarky thing I said about the First Classes (the consequences of COVID had not settled in as a deadly reality because we were so isolated from the rest of civilization). Multiply that by 78 people and I think at the end of it there were over 1,000 pieces of mail distributed by HM3 Ho Vo and his team of comrades.

11 April 2020
Day 53 & 54

There is a reason why my favorite number is 54. Well, the literal reason is because my 9th grade head football coach assigned me that number. I remember feeling so special, like I was the chosen one who would bring glory to the number. Little did I know that it would only last two seasons, and a guy in the year behind me, Eric, would take my number away from me because I was late to join the team. Not going to get into specifics, but it wasn't my idea to keep me off the team. When I did come on the team my junior year, I was #63, and I quit halfway through the season. It's funny, looking back on it, I don't exactly remember why I quit, like what was the final straw. I hope I wrote that down somewhere else.

Anyway, let it be known that on the 54th day since leaving Japan the announcement came that we'd be traveling together to Afghanistan. Word around the campfire is we're leaving April 22. If that is in fact true, I'll be able to sigh a bit of relief because I have a lot of stuff coming in the mail from soap, to stamps, envelopes, my Chromebook, mouse, and batteries. Everything should arrive by the 15th.

I'm jazzed about the stamps because they are Hot Wheels themed and I'm excited to start mailing them to the boys. Oh, I almost bought a box of the pens I prefer and a couple more journals because this one is probably going to only take me out to 100 days. I'm thankful to HN Kevin Pham, and considered asking that he send more, but what I'm writing in is a gift, not a requirement. His generosity at Christmas was enough.

From within the night the COVID-19 stimulus relief stipend came in. It was an extra $3,400 Saori was not expecting. I absolutely hate telling her we're expecting money to come in because she has the patience of—wait, she has no chill when it comes to getting paid. Plus, this way I can surprise her with something.

I spent a good deal of this morning cleaning the armory and reading my book. Yes, I'm still on the Laura Ingalls Wilder biography. It's okay, not what I expected. I find myself so much more productive when the phone is turned off, or at least when the Wi-Fi is.

Last night I finished watching *The New Pope* (2019). I remember seeing the trailer wondering how they were going to pull that off, inserting Malkovich while retaining Jude Law, but they did in splendid fashion. I enjoyed the second season more than the first.

Yesterday we had pizza delivered to us, and I was a gluttonous little piggy. I have decided to transcribe my deployment journal onto Google Docs. From there I don't know what I'll do with it. Caffeine gives me too many ideas to tackle. Gotta focus.

Postscript: I immediately bought the soundtrack to The New Pope *because I was that impressed by the musical selection. Leaving together was great news, but it became a hilariously anxious time because I really wanted my stuff to arrive in the mail before I shipped out. From time to time I write and include in the transcribed version about writing in my actual journal from the grip of the pens to the amount of paper. I always thought it important for the reader to know that this was all done by hand at one point.*

14 April 2020
Day 56 & 57

What a day or two filled with peculiar problems. There is so much input on things I want to do, but I'm quite simply overloaded. From the top, *House M.D.* (2004) is on Amazon Prime. Although I've mentioned this before, I feel like I must binge through until the end. I gave it the old college try last night, and this was the first day in Texas I woke up tired. To give an idea how popular that show was, there were eight seasons with 22 episodes per season. No wonder why actors get burnt out playing the same roles.

Next, my Chromebook arrived in the mail yesterday. There is clearly a lot to do on it especially pertaining to Google Docs. I need to get over my writer's block for *Opie & The Foreman*, transcribe this journal, and anything else that comes to mind. I added a screenwriting app last night; I need to nut up or shut up when it comes to sitting there and doing creative work. Also, my pens and envelopes came in the mail so I can start writing letters again.

This has me pretty jazzed up, but again, it takes time. There is a lot of progress in my L.I. Wilder book too. I'm more than halfway, finally, and pledged to myself, in an effort to have less YouTube time, to read 50 pages a day. Yesterday was my first day, and with everything else in mind I don't know if this will keep up. In spurts, probably.

Then there is the YouTube podcast review of *The New Pope* (2019). Each episode is almost as long, if not longer than the actual show, so in essence I'm watching the season over again.

Of course, I need time for the track. I think I've been doing a good job on limiting my meals. Also, I've added some jogging and squats. Most ideally, I can get out there twice a day for a total of six miles, but because of the wind I'm just making excuses for myself to go once. Today is my rest day.

When I'm outside I like my audiobook. It's called *Working Stiff* and it's about a pathological medical examiner. There's enough terminology to make me feel elitist but dumbed down enough for me to fully understand. Good pace and stories about a field I really haven't given much thought.

So, the latest word is April 26 is the fly-out date. Outstanding.

Postscript: I loved watching House, *and completing the series was a fine moment for me, but more on that later. Around this time, the tempo began to pick up, and consequently it required me to be more productive with my mind. I now had the tools to complete my goals, but the excuses remained. I understood what Hemingway said about making the paper bleed but putting it into actual practice seemed so daunting for some reason. I felt like a dog running up to a lake. How fun it would be to just dive in, but the unfamiliar caused plenty of hesitation. I recognized that, and it was another mental hurdle.*

15 April 2020
Day 58

It's the 26th year after my father's death. Like normal, I shared a few words with my mom and sister, Rachael. Not much more to say about that.

Possibly the funniest story about being the supply bitch happened today. The Executive Officer, Captain Jeff Klinger, came to my room with Senior Chief asking me to get base facilities to turn off the air-conditioning of the building NEXT to us. Why? Because it was too loud and became a distraction. Of course, I put in the request, and I'm just happy I have such a good rapport with them. Still, they laughed in my face. Still more, the sound had disappeared, and I looked like the hero by McGregor standards.

I've taken a nap and now I'm pretty jazzed up to rework the *Opie & The Foreman* outline. I'd really like to get back to work.

Our Lean Six Sigma course is really starting to build steam, and that is cool, but I have other things on my burners that are also important. I do understand, however, that professionally this is a big deal to me, and the timeline is set by someone else. Would prove wise to get on their program because this is an opportunity I've been waiting for.

One thing I am most fortunate for is that I am never bored. My promise to God remains upheld.

Postscript: My promise to God remains upheld. In boot camp there is not a lot of individuality. In fact, it is highly frowned upon. During the first few days of processing, we wake up very early in the morning and head to medical where we are examined by dental and immunizations, and everything else to start a Sailor out on their journey. There is a lot of waiting around, standing, and sitting in a line. We were not allowed to sleep at all. It was then I made a promise to God that if he got me through this, I would never be bored again. Since those days, I have never thought of myself as bored and always found something to do, to think about, to improve, or work on. It may not have been the right thing to do, but I never thought of myself as bored. The story with Captain Klinger was absolutely ridiculous, and he had to have known it, but idle minds lead to wandering lawful orders. This was a casualty of that. Not sure how the air-conditioning ever got fixed though.

18 April 2020
Day 59, 60 & 61

Yet another laundry day for the Sconnie Sailor. The past couple of days have been both interesting and routine. We are supposed to have a sandstorm starting in a couple hours. It's 0935 and the wind is relatively calm now, but then again it normally is in the morning hours. This will be my first sandstorm, so I'm curious to see what it's like. No one is panicking or going into TCCOR (Tropical Cyclone Conditions of Readiness) conditions.

This *House M.D.* (2004) on Amazon Prime has a firm grip on my priorities. I'm a quarter of the way finished with season six. Some episodes are familiar, but I can't remember if I saw them or if they are clips from the internet.

The other day I penned a letter to Brandon Wydra, but I didn't have a stamp. I wanted to pay for postage by weight instead, but the post office staff was so kind to me. They took a 55-cent stamp of their own to use on my letter. I was so appreciative I took the time to write them an ICE, or Interactive Customer Evaluation, comment.

Yesterday, I received an email that my two books of Hot Wheel stamps were shipped. Only six days after placing the order. I'll blame not a lot of essential workers at the United States Postal Service headquarters. Today I think I want to write to my friend Robert, and if I don't get around to it today then I most definitely will soon enough. Besides, there is no mail service on the weekends at McGregor Range anyway.

One of my added jobs at supply/facilities is to issue out the gun cases for when we travel. It's a slow process, but I think it's meant to be that way. Part of the method behind the madness. One might say that it's getting me a lot of face time with everyone. I'm going to enjoy not having to do this job when we leave here.

Had a very nice conversation with Dr. Solomon yesterday. We talk about many things, but today in particular was about writing. She said something that really piqued my interest in that "although writing is a linear product, it is a circular process." I think that is why I'm spending so much time now on the outline.

It did pain me mildly, however, at the sobering realization that I will most likely be tweaking my outline a few times throughout the process.

Captain Dan Kahler wants to learn about Chromebooks today. I'm excited.

Which leads me to the thing I love to complain about the most, *The Whiskey Ration* and the PAO. It was released yesterday and there was more to be desired. For starters, the rest of the team had one evening to review and provide input. The rest of the team gave a quick greenlight. There was incorrect grammar, misspelled words, and irresponsible programs and initiatives. I will always wonder how people decide what is important to them. I'm treating this newsletter like it's my last stand. Why though? It is incredibly frustrating to a productive and industrious Second Class. When will my time come? How long must I wait? What must I do to stop this cycle?

So, I wrote an email intended for the PAO team, but directed at LCDR Fitzgerald. When I finished, I could sense it was too personal. I shared it with Senior Chief Wink, Chief Atanagan, HM1 Wilson, and Captain Kahler. They all said I made excellent points, which is good. I'm not trying to replace anyone as the PAO. What I want is to be included on the team. Taken seriously, and not be included in bad decisions without the chance to announce my objection first. Big asks, I know. Such drama.

Postscript: That email was full of cringe when looking back on it. No one treated the newsletter like it was a precious document like I did. What did that email prove except that I was being a top-tier douchebag without an ounce of trying to be a team player? At the time, I honestly thought I was doing the right thing to keep the ship from sinking, but in reality, I was jettisoning my leadership capital by making more problems than actually existed. At least I was aware of my own disruption to my tranquility when talking about the PAO program. Although I'm not at the desired levels, to become self-aware is an important quality.

19 April 2020
Day 62

Yesterday's "sandstorm" was a dud. There was nothing to write about except that it was so underwhelming. We did not have muster today because it was Sunday. I still had to wake up at 0730 to text HM1 Wilson that I wasn't dead. Then I fell back asleep for a couple of hours and was out of bed by 1000.

Saw Captain Kahler shaving as I took my morning trip to the urinal, and he asked what I had planned today. I told him, to write. I had to struggle watching the end of *Jumanji 2: The Next Level* (2019). The best part was Kevin Hart's and The Rock's impressions of Danny Glover and Danny DeVito respectively. Besides that, I was not on board with the film, no pun intended.

Now I'm in the computer lab where there is an empty desk, and I'm happier than a deck seaman on payday. Except the part where they are pretty serious about wearing a mask.

Later today I have watch, so I'll have more time for other stuff. The amount of time isn't the problem, it's the dedication spent on devoting that time wisely and not to piss it away.

Postscript: We all knew our time to leave was getting close, and it was an antsy time for everyone. Although details were still murky, we could feel the new dawn beginning to shine upon our faces.

20 April 2020
Day 63

Today could have gone better. It started with a headache, which lasted through most of the day. Our Wi-Fi went out for a portion of the day, too. It was DCSS's day to serve food. In all, I mostly tried to sleep and feel sorry for myself.

Not everything was bad, however. My stamps finally arrived, and I mailed out the letter to my friend Robert. I also mailed the card that was returned to me destined for the boys and women of Arita.

We also had a meeting with the PAO team. I felt it went well, we used my pre-meeting notes as the agenda. Now that I have the reins of the newsletter, it has been delegated to the enlisted, this is my cross to carry. I just hope my mouth can write checks my ass will be able to cash.

Because the internet was late coming on, I was late to call Saori. The boys are staying home from daycare, and they were watching TV, which doesn't bother me until Saori says they watch too much TV. I had my shirt off in front of her, and I know I didn't look like any progress was made. She made some little comment, and it took care of the rest of the conversation. So yes, today I didn't feel very good about me.

Postscript: My headaches are normally induced by two factors, not having my glasses and stress. Since masks were not standard yet, I rocked my glasses with that thick black strap to keep them in place. This was one of the reasons why I was Captain Kahler's "son," because he had the same strap for his glasses. When it came to serving food, we had vans that would drive out to the DFAC to pick up big vats of food that hardly anyone ate from because it was the same meal every three days or so: chicken, chili mac, or something else gross. We could not return the food, so we ended up wasting so much food every day. They would give up loaves of bread, boxes of jelly and peanut butter, and cases of fruit every day. Most of it went to waste. This ended up being a familiar scene once we got to Afghanistan that is written more about later.

21 April 2020
Day 64

I can't believe yesterday was 4/20 and almost literally no one cared, just what I like to see. It is stupid to celebrate smoking weed, or at least dedicate an entire day to it.

Today we got the word, we fly out on the 26th. Since the flight is leaving at 0900, we're going to be up and rocking by 0300. It's going to be a long day, but everyone is excited. I think it feels a little surreal, like wow, this is actually happening. As the facilities petty officer for these two crack houses, I'm getting fired up. There is a lot to do in my mind's eye. Hopefully with enough teamwork it will all go fine.

Besides that, I don't believe I did a lot. There were a few entries of this journal transcribed onto the computer, and I finished handing out the weapons cases. All except one, LCDR Tom Warner. I don't know if he has forgotten or if he's playing games with me. He'll eventually need the case.

Had a good conversation with LCDR Krystel Salazar. We talked about human logic and how we are flawed. We also talked about cultured systems and the differences between Asian and American norms specifically.

I finished season six of *House M.D.* (2004); only 2 more to go. Called my mom; well, she called me. It was okay; we talked about nurses.

Postscript: There should be an entire sub-chapter on nurses here. It always seemed like no one was fine with saying they were just a nurse but would go out of their way telling me what kind of nurse. Flight nurse, ICU nurse, trauma nurse, it was like their identity hung on their specialty. Smoking marijuana has always been a polarizing subject for me. Although today I consider myself moderately progressive, there was a time I left romantic relationships because we could not agree on how we viewed the culture. It helped me realign my position when my friend said that he never knew anyone who beat their wife while high. There is a pharmacy joke that there is better living through chemistry. If it helps relieve pain and promote a higher quality of life, then there is a place for it. Like any drug however, it can be abused, and it can also ruin lives. It can rob someone of potential, but so can alcohol. Moderation and self-awareness are important factors to consider if it is right for you.

23 April 2020
Days 65 & 66

Only a couple days to go before we ship out. What to do in the time prior. The Wi-Fi is out so I'm left with plenty of opportunity to catch up on writing.

While doing laundry this morning, instead of inputting my entries, I wrote letters instead. In today's case I wrote to Master Chief Lorenzo Branch, Senior Enlisted Leader of BHC Sasebo, and to HN Kevin Pham. They were about two separate topics; as it should be, I think. To Pham it was about encouragement and staying the course. To Master Chief it was about my fears and concerns.

One letter was harder to write, Master Chief's. Before writing to him, we were asked if we should want to extend if given the choice. It was a hard decision, much worse than jumping onto this deployment to begin with, but I volunteered myself to be extended. Saori will never know I willingly stepped forward to stay away longer than initially planned. I wish we didn't have a choice to be extended. That's what my letter was about, trying to explain why I made this choice.

In essence, I said I don't know what it takes to be a First Class, but I'm desperate and will do what I need to in order to reach career security. I tried to make it about me and not drag others into it. My hope is he reads the intent and the purity of the message.

Now I know what Maynard James Keenan from Tool meant in his song "10,000 Days" when he said that "10,000 days in the fire" and "it's my time now, my time now…" What more do I need to do?

Yesterday was a little bit more positive. We completed our Lean Six Sigma Green Belt course. I guess technically we need to start working on our two projects to earn the NEC (Navy Enlisted Classification).

All gun cases are now issued, and that makes me feel good. From the sounds of it, Qatar sounds like it's going to suck, but we won't be in

Texas, and to me that's all that matters. We had another trivia night yesterday, too. We won a round, but another team took two rounds for the overall win. I'm slightly hooked on a new phone app; it's "Who Wants to be a Millionaire?" I'm almost halfway done with season seven of *House M.D.* (2004). Will finish it off while in KAF.

Josey finished an 80-piece puzzle in one day.

Postscript: In all the times I have spent either writing to Master Chief Branch or in his office, he has only made one reference to the existence of my letters. That is a kind of leadership I hope to better understand. I'm about recognizing those attempts to better connect. He certainly read what I had to say, but as we will see later on, writing a letter has become a lost art, and I'm glad I can still carry the torch. Josiah has an impeccable memory. We will go to a Japanese bath house (called an onsen) maybe one time and he'll remember it. Like most children I'm sure, he's always surprising his parents with what he knows.

24 April 2020
Day 67

Almost, just maybe, I'm feeling rushed. After weeks being in wait, it's starting to happen, the realization that we're leaving. I have begun to pack, sort of. Honestly, I'm dragging my feet.

Today I wrote my last letter while in Texas. It was to Zach Nebus. Because of my output of letters, and uncertainty that the recipients are keeping my letters, I've dropped from the traditional three pages to two.

Also today, we had a cookout to celebrate us leaving here. Never would I ever have imagined that I would appreciate the taste of a cheap hamburger. I had two. Went back to my room and "tried" to take a nap, but it was so damn hot that I was just miserable. Why we don't turn the air-conditioning on in south Texas in late April is beyond me. Each night lately is miserable. Only two more nights to go.

I started listening to the new Jim Ross book *Beyond the Black Hat.* So far, it's good. Sat down with HM3 James Writer to discuss the newsletter. Excellent meeting. I was able to lay out my guidance and expectations, and I got to hear his. It will be a good issue.

Working outside tonight. It's too hot in my room.

Postscript: The toilet paper closet that I had made my room was in the same hallway as the oldest officers of the deployment. Not to mention the Senior Enlisted Advisor, Executive Officer, Commanding Officer, Chief of Surgery, and Chief of Medicine (among other notables) were all stacked one after another from my room. There little HM2 Rastall was, sweating and complaining, but as they say, a bitching Sailor is a happy Sailor [because it means they still have hope]. The air-conditioning was turned off in my hallway, and I seriously considered either moving back into my original assigned room with two other guys or accept that getting chewed out was the best course of action by turning on the air with one swift unilateral decision. I chose neither and decided to just complain more about it in my journal.

SPADES

Although I cannot speak for every branch of military service, I will say with authority that the Navy has an unofficial game amongst the Sailors. When you're not playing Bones (dominos), you are probably playing Spades. Even if you don't play Spades, you better know how to play. It will either become cause for much ridicule or get yourself labeled as a boot.

In my own Spades journey I considered myself fortunate because my introduction happened at such a tender age. Way back in Hospital Corps School, or "A" school at the one true location, Great Lakes, IL, (it has since moved to Fort Sam Houston, TX) near the end of the class, I was able to watch some classmates play our instructors. What piqued my interest the most about all of this was everyone knew how to play a game that up until that point I had never heard of. It was also a small window of time when military good order and discipline was set aside for obtaining the competitive edge necessary to getting inside your opponent's head, which I have come to understand is an important element to success.

Our head instructor was HMC James Wallace. He said three things that stuck with me. The first was about his name. He always introduced himself as "Chief Wallace, with two Ls." I always found that funny in a way because I couldn't think of another way to spell Wallace with just one L. The second reason I found it amusing was my last name had a double consonant, and since that day I use it too. It's Cal Rastall, with two Ls. Only the joke was on me because people still mess it up and forget the second L.

Second thing about Chief was about haircuts. In school I got my haircut every two weeks, and it was always on a Sunday, so I'd be looking fresh for work the next morning. Because I always liked short hair, I told the barber the only hairstyle I knew, "high and tight." The next day I'm at work and I fail an exam, so it is required I go to remedial study, a room separate from the classroom where you're able to relearn something you should have taken seriously days before like the rest of your classmates. At this point in the course, I didn't even know if I wanted to be a Hospital Corpsman let alone stay in a student status where you're treated above a boot camp resident, but less than a fleet Sailor. I went to remedial study and was giving the First Class Petty Officer a hard time by being snarky and mildly disrespectful. In boot camp it is acceptable to call any Petty Officer just that, but in "A" School you are expected to know their rating, and in this case, I was not giving this First Class the respect of calling her "HM1." Little did I know that becoming a First Class, or E-6, would be as hard for me as it was easy to look down upon her at the time. So, she asked me who my Chief was, and I said, "HMC Wallace with two Ls" with full conviction believing that he'd come in and save the day. Again, I was wrong. It was my first real ass-chewing outside of boot camp, and he undressed me like nothing I'd ever heard before. He was a smoker at the time, and he got really close to my face and asked me if I was ever going to get a haircut "you hippie." I'll remind you that I had just gotten a high and tight literally the day before. I wasn't sure if I was going to stay in school let alone stay in the Navy after that one-way conversation. Needless to say, it got me straight in a hurry.

The third thing about Chief Wallace, with two Ls, was he would always say that he'd never become a Senior Chief because he didn't play the game. Fast forward seven years and I'm stationed in Branch Health Clinic Iwakuni, Japan. Because the stars aligned just right, I needed to take my advancement exam in Madison, WI, while I was on leave. That was coordinated through the reserve center, which was run by the Chicago Recruiting District. This type of request is first funneled through the Command Master Chief, and you wouldn't guess who it was, CMDCM James Wallace. To give some context, in seven years, he not only made it up to Master Chief, but a level above Master Chief to Command Master Chief. The funny thing was he remembered me and sent his best.

Back to playing Spades with Chief and the fleet returnee Sailors hoping to become Corpsman, some of the things that were said were quite saucy and there wasn't a knife hand to be seen. I really admired that and convinced myself that this was a game I had to learn how to play.

Jump ahead to my time on the USS Theodore Roosevelt (CVN 71), and we are playing spades: my LPO, a prior-enlisted doctor who was a submariner, and the physical therapist. We played in the biggest space available outside of causing a scene, in the physical therapist's office. Being the low man on the totem pole, I set the game up, got boxes and chairs together, but the prize for winning the game was not having to put it all back. This was high stakes in a cash-free zone. My partner was my LPO, and we ended up winning, but not without me saying things that would make Davy Jones cringe. I'm hooting and hollering in celebration just laying into these officers because that was the spirit of Spades. The physical therapist, a straight up officer, never received that memo, and said straight to me, "I'm not picking that shit up, you are." It was at that point I knew I wanted to leave the Navy. The next day I submitted my request to take the Transition Assistance Program and prepare for separation from the Navy. I was so mad I didn't care what it would cost me, if I didn't need to take orders from the worst officer I ever met in my life or anyone of her kind. My Departmental Leading Chief Petty Officer, Senior Chief Greg Fall, led me up to the hangar bay and in a way that only he could, got me down from my tower of fury and led me to a decision I was going to make all along, reenlist.

Now we are in McGregor, and I'm playing against officers again. My teammate, HM2 Chris Parchmon, is just running house, and I'm well inside the minds of my opponents, a couple of Lieutenants. Well, one at least, and she let me have it. Instead of wanting to separate from the Navy, the economics of that were just too outside of acceptable, I decided to become mad at the Lieutenant, who was prior enlisted, and some unnecessary bad blood was formed out there on the table. When that story made it into the first issue of *The Thirsty Camel*, all became well, and the animosity was put to rest.

Spades have played a very important part of my life throughout my time in the Navy. It rates its own substory and I'm happy to share it. Too many movies show poker as the game of choice, and that is disheartening to see. Oh, that physical therapist? She was promoted and became the Department Head at a big west coast hospital and was the boss of the physical therapist on the deployment. Small Navy, still the worst officer I ever worked for, and was once the sole reason why I was going to leave it all behind.

25 April 2020
Day 68

Technically it is 0320 on April 26, but my day on the 25th never really ended, because I have yet to go to sleep.

For some reason I woke up for breakfast, which was strange. That normally never happens. When we began to pack, I think the worst part for me was separating my personal responsibilities with professional. In many ways I was not crisp and efficient with my preparedness. Of course, I snuck in one more nap, but it wasn't so long.

I wish I had one more seabag so everything would comfortably fit, but we can't all be so fortunate. It was strange, the tempo picked up after dinner, yet there was plenty of hurrying up to wait.

At last, the final inspection came at 0030 and it happened, we were cleared to leave McGregor Range. It was a surreal feeling, driving past the gates. Now we sit at the plane terminal waiting to board. The luggage loading crew is loading the plane now. I did not volunteer for this task because I feel like I have pulled enough weight as the supply/facilities guy.

Now I just want Senior Chief Wink to ceremoniously fire me and relieve me of these duties so I can breathe.

Postscript: This entire deployment was full of expectations being subverted. The joke was yet again played on me. Not only was I not ceremoniously fired, but I was somehow still tagged as the supply guy in Qatar. I was still relieved to leave McGregor, a place I hope I will never have to return to again, but I have no doubt I will one day need to return.

28 April 2020
Days 69, 70 & 71

How much could change in such a short amount of time? Well, Whiskey Rotation dared to find out. It started with waiting at the El Paso Airport for three hours. Chief Gillette gave me a couple going away gifts as tokens of his appreciation, including phone cards, imported Japanese bottled green tea, a gun cleaning kit, and a 5" k-bar knife. I didn't open the bag until after we parted ways with our checked luggage. HM2 Jesse John thought he could get the k-bar into his checked luggage but was unsuccessful. My only two options were to somehow get the knife through airport security or to give it back to Chief Gillette and ask him to forward it in the mail. As luck would have it, and there was plenty to go around these past few days, I ran into Chief one last time before boarding. The weird part was our luggage went totally unchecked from El Paso to Qatar. It was the most bizarre airport experience ever. Hopefully Chief will mail it so I can take it on hikes against the wild boars.

It was a 2.5-hour flight to somewhere in Georgia where we picked up an Air Force unit. It was about a two-hour layover, and we had Dominos delivered for lunch. It was back on the same plane for an 8.5-hour flight to the Frankfurt/Hahn Airport. It felt like a two-hour flight because Benadryl is a heck of a drug.

That brings us to Germany. First of all, it looks a lot like Wisconsin, but no surprise there if we pause to think about that. The weather was cool and dewy, and it was 0550 when we touched down. The Commanding Officer authorized alcohol and reminded us to be "responsible adults." Some Sailors had a reputation to uphold, and the high score I heard amongst us over the two-hour layover was 11 beers. I didn't drink, although I did find it interesting beer cost the same as soda. What I told people, and there is truth, is although I'm not a problem when I drink, once the fun starts it's hard for me to stop, and that *is* a problem. Maybe the real truth is I'm not comfortable enough with anyone yet to drink with them.

Then the fun started. It was a six-hour flight to Qatar from Germany. I didn't eat anything; I wasn't hungry. When we parked in Qatar, an air crew guy boarded, let us know it was over 100 degrees and he needed 15 volunteers to help unload the plane. If I learned anything in Texas, it was that the Navy stood for Never Again Volunteer Yourself. It was mostly the Air Force and one of our own guys, HM2 Wilbon Robinson.

I get bloated while flying, and I can do a good job finding a toilet to let out the air and anything else built up. We were herded up, had to walk a quarter mile (hot), and forced to stand in line for processing. They had porta-potties, and I misjudged that final fart. Luckily, I was wearing underwear, but still had to wipe more than I wanted to in a tiny porta-potty.

I was miserable, my first night in Qatar was textbook hurry-up-and-wait. We didn't leave the airport until six hours after arriving. It is also the middle of Ramadan here, which didn't help anyone. There was no work to be done before sunset. I had atomic toilet episodes two more times; just so much gas built up, it was the worst.

So we finally got out to lodging. It was a textbook cluster. They were like, "Pair with your roommate." I was one of the final people to get a room because I never had a roommate in Texas. At the time, I would have been glad to live with anyone, but somehow a miracle was done, and I was assigned a room to myself. It didn't have a fridge or power converter, but at the time I didn't care.

Was finally asleep at 0200. My paranoid mind was up at 0615. One thing about the Qatari night/morning is the breeze and temperature are most agreeable. The morning trip to the urinal included me crapping my pants again. This time with no underwear. I took my second shower in four hours and vowed never to trust myself again.

The days are hot, I took two grams of Tylenol with hardly a dent of headache relief. Food from the galley is good so far. There is a lot of napping, and we need to get our temperature checked twice a day. Woke up at 2145, sat outside, and prayed about a lot of things. Walked back inside to find a bag of laundry pods. I did a load of my soiled clothes and sat down to finally write.

Postscript: This entry made it into The Whiskey Ration *as an article. It was almost submitted verbatim, but I never read the final product once it finished the line of editing. I was miserable, but we were not in America, so that was cool. For the next two weeks we stayed in another quarantine environment before finally settling down in the CENTCOM, or Central Command region.*

29 April 2020
Day 72

Another disclosed technicality, but it's 0315 on April 30. I am definitely jetlagged, and right now I'm okay with that. The nights are so nice. For the past three evenings there has been a nice breeze, and my skin isn't feeling like it's in a convection oven like it does during the day.

Of course, a day cannot be complete without some drama. Some of us, myself included, jumped ahead of our designated time to eat breakfast. We have different color wristbands between what's called "cohorts." The idea is to group us together to limit exposure from other units. It's all a joke, even Senior Chief said so, but later in the day he had to message us three times about it. I almost feel bad for him about this, but it makes me consider the other mountains of adversity he, and Chiefs in general, must endure. As Chief Matt Struble once told me, they have to come out as a unified front once a decision has been made.

I finished season seven of *House M.D.* (2004) and am now on the final lap. I might just open my laptop after this because God knows I haven't cracked open my book yet. Been too busy with adjusting and not being bored with other stimulants first.

Might call Japan too. They are six hours in front of us. Was invited to work out by LT Byrd too, so I will probably fail big time. I need to.

Postscript: We stayed in these long trailer looking buildings that from what I was told, were scheduled to be condemned prior to the COVID outbreak. I didn't really want to touch anything in my room and always made sure to wear shower sandals rather than walking barefoot. There was a communal bathroom where everyone could shower and use the toilets, but we stayed on the other end of the trailer barracks.

30 April 2020
Day 73

Still jet lagged, but as it's already established, I am okay with that. I reek of Icy Hot balm right now. I'm very sore from working out with LT Byrd this morning. We did a half-Kolten the Terrible; my time was 44:14. We did 25 lunges, pushups, squats, flutter kicks, and burpees. Second set would be 20, third 15, etc. to 5 reps on the final set. Well, for the burpees, I stopped at 10 and only did 10 until the last set. I was fried.

After PT, we went to breakfast after showering. I was slow. Then crawled into bed to watch *House*. I'm on episode 10 of 23. There really wasn't too much more to my day. The past two days we experienced a real sandstorm. It wasn't epic, but you could hear the wind howl and visibility was affected.

Had another interesting conversation with LCDR Krystel Salazar. We spoke a while about how I asked questions and down the rabbit hole we went. We got to talking about capitalism. I don't know why she engaged me, I'm sitting alone on this picnic table, but I'm glad she did. I don't exactly get the chance to talk to many people since I don't have a roommate. I'll say it again for emphasis, there is a big difference between solitude and loneliness.

Chief Ringpis contacted me today. No doubt out of obligation because of the NFAAS (Navy Family Accountability and Assessment System) notification. Miss my kids and working.

Postscript: It cannot be understated how hot it was. I had never experienced anything like it in my life. Although I did a good job staying out of the sun for the most part, there were some situations that could not be helped. For example, the meals. We were supposed to eat according to our cohort schedule, but that was clearly an initiative that looked good on paper but was awful when applied. The food lines could not keep up with the amount of people who wanted to eat causing delays. Then they tried to enforce social distancing, which didn't work because that would have backed the line up around the compound. When you weren't in line to eat during the day, you slept, but if you had to use the bathroom, you had to go outside and be blasted with a hellish wave of heat. It was so hot they had pallets upon pallets of bottled water just waiting for you to take. They never rationed the water, and you always made sure to have at least 12 bottles in the fridge.

1 May 2020
Day 74

These days I think it's better to talk a little each day about nothing than save up across multiple days to talk about nothing.

My days are bleak, but I am not bored. That makes sense in my mind. My sleep pattern remains pleasantly jacked up. I'm up all night; I tell myself it's the time to be productive when all I'm really doing is slaying *House M.D.* (2004) episodes. I should be completing the series tomorrow. I'm excited because I've been blaming a lot of my non-productivity on *House*. Looking back on it I can say that I maintained an incredible pace.

When I finish this entry, I will open the Chromebook and get cracking on the newsletter. Not only was it on my agenda today anyway, but both LT Simon Prado and HM3 Ho Vo on separate occasions had questions regarding the update on the newsletter. It's good that everyone is still caring and holds one another accountable.

Oh! I was accused of going to the "real" galley not for quarantined personnel. They were so certain too but played it off as a cautionary tale. Although there are some stupid rules here, some we know not to break such as getting caught outside the fence line.

PT with LT Byrd beat me down again today. I'm sorer than I was yesterday. I found out the hard way that Icy Hot does not feel good close to the armpits.

Postscript: For the common folk out here reading, PT is military-speech for Physical Training, or working out. Besides being blessed with my own room, I was fortunate, along with everyone else, to have access to the internet while in Qatar. Some sites were blocked unless you used a VPN, which I had, but other than that I didn't necessarily need to be in a room by myself. By this time, I was feeling very detached from everyone else.

2 May 2020
Day 75

Has it really been 75 days since saying goodbye to Japan? In perspective we aren't even halfway into deployment yet. The day was once again scorching hot. Luckily, I didn't hardly go outside, except to use the restroom after waking up. I did go to breakfast which has begun to sadly lose its appeal. When that joy leaves, I'm going to be in trouble. It's too hot to walk to the chow hall, but I'll need to eat. At least with lunch and dinner there is variety. With breakfast it's the same thing except a change in cereal selection.

I cannot remember ever being this sore. My lats, ribs, buttocks, and chest hurt the most. It's literally sensitive to the touch. Luckily LT Byrd was like, "Weekends we don't do anything." Thank goodness. I was more sore yesterday than the two days prior combined. Just looking forward to the misery to pass so I can start to excel.

As promised, I finished *House M.D.* (2004) today. The last episode was mildly controversial. I feel he should have stayed dead and brought back Cuddy for the finale. Plus, the writing was all over the place with loopholes and it was just inconclusive. Maybe there are parallels to how *Sherlock Holmes* ended, but maybe I will let this lie.

After waking up, I did start to feel better. Started tying Issue #2 together. Sent out emails for reminders and will prep my interview questions tonight. Will also need to review Lean Six Sigma paperwork. Fun.

Postscript: I don't think I'll ever forget my time in Qatar. Being caged in, gun decking our temperatures with thermometers that didn't work, being burned alive. One of the interesting parts was the picnic table outside of our trailer. It was commandeered by Whiskey Sailors during the day, and they'd all sit around this little table and people watch in the heat of the day. Because the trailers were supposed to be condemned, many were abandoned, which led to interesting finds by the Whiskey scout HM2 Jesse John. He found all sorts of things; among them was a tactical tarp he rigged to use as an awning for everyone to sit beneath.

3 May 2020
Day 76

Called Baraboo for the first time since getting to Qatar. Talked to my mother for the longest time, 87 minutes. It was a real good conversation, and I learned some things. My folks have been jettisoning stuff for years since they became empty nesters. I asked her what was so important about a rocking chair that had been carted across America a couple of times. It was so plain, and I have pondered for a while what the appeal has been in keeping it across the years. She told me it was the first new piece of furniture she ever bought, and that was something I learned about my mother today.

Wrote an article by the Sconnie Sailor today for the newsletter. I'm looking forward to revising it tonight. Had an in-person conversation with LCDR Fitzgerald. She called me out on me having a problem with her and not being quiet about it. I'm glad she did that, and although I didn't state my grievances right there (I had literally just woken up from a nap and was taken by surprise), it does open the door in the future. Most likely this will be addressed again.

Looking forward to working out again and the soreness has gone away considerably. Saori and I did get into a little fight about money today. She means well, but there is a bad combination of anxiety and boredom on my end. Something to work on.

Postscript: Yes, the typical spousal argument. I have no idea what the fight was about even after rereading this entry. No doubt it was just to take up dead space in the conversation. Because I was literally doing nothing, she only had enough strength from her days to answer the same kinds of questions: "how are the boys," "how is your mom," "what's the weather like?" I'm really glad LCDR Fitzgerald confronted me because I was too chicken shit to do it myself.

4 May 2020
Day 77

May the Fourth be with you. Everyone always talks about "Star Wars Day," but few and far between do I see people celebrate it. This journal entry is not what this is about though. I slept from 1100 to temperature checks at 1600, looked at my watch at 1730 to realize I wasn't going to make it to dinner, slept more until about 2030, was awake but tossed and turned in bed, then finally woke up at 0230 on May 5.

What I chose to dream about and the reason I dreamt what I did is the most haunting. A great deal of my evening was spent trying to chase my first love from high school, a girl who I used to know. We have each moved on from one another; she is now married and has a child of her own. We hadn't spoken in years. Why tonight and why her? There were plenty of bad memories, some of which I am not proud of at all, but my dream felt like I was chasing my youth.

Those electric nights of being young and in love. It felt like I was in the Toby Keith song "Dream Walking." Whenever I thought it'd be quiet and just us, something would happen to disrupt the entire evening. I wasn't even talking about wanting sex with her one last time, but to share a moment of a simpler time in my life. Some of my best memories of my budding years were with her, and I'm happy I dreamt of her. I'm even more happy we did not last and that Saori and my sons are the bulk of my life instead. I doubt that she thinks of me anymore and that's okay. I dreamt of being young and it was a magical feeling.

Postscript: The reality of the dream was that it was jolting and snapped me awake. I meant every word I wrote, and it makes me wonder if I will dream about being young more often the older I get. I'm on the back nine of my career in the Navy, and it feels like I'm surrounded by people who are at an age where I could physically be their parent. I suppose that is a feeling I should start getting used to, especially in the Navy.

PRISON GYM

I've said it once, and it'll be said many more times, I don't like lifting weights. Slinging the iron and that culture is not the life I'm about. What I am all for, is seeing creativity and watching something magical happen because of it. Who knew meatheads could be so ingenious, but there I was left in awe once again.

Qatar was a flat, deserted desert. The compound we were in was fenced to keep us separated from the general population. This in turn made us creative when it came to physical training. I was perfectly fine with bodyweight exercises. The typical pushups, crunches, and burpees. Believe me, there was plenty of weight to lift. Then there were the guys who were destined to become as creative as possible when it came to lifting weights.

I coined it the prison gym because it had the most ratchet pieces of "equipment" that could be mustered. They would find a pvc pipe, put two cinder blocks on each end, and suddenly you were capable of a bench press, curl press, squat, or deadlift. The guys would take turns recording themselves doing these ridiculous exercises and then share it with the rest of Whiskey Rotation.

There were of course the regulars who never missed an opportunity to lift. Among them were HM1 Jake Wilson, HM1 Jake Kubil, and HM2 Jed Rodriguez. Then there were the supporting characters who would join in every now and again, but were not the hardliners, HM2 Nicholas Slagle, HN Clarissa Dreadin, and HM3 Harlie Valdez.

The PT groups in Qatar were more separated than that. There was a group that was all about tabata classes. These maniacs were possibly the largest group, and they were always and consistently out there. I didn't want to expose myself in peer groups like this, which I now know was contradictory to the entire point, so I personally worked out with LT Byrd. He would do a workout with me, send me limping back to my room, then catch a lift session with the other reservist officers.

We had a group of walkers, generally the older population, who would get lapped by the Director for Administration, also known as DFA, who was the Energizer Bunny of the Rotation. People tried to match him, but he kept an incredible pace with no one to rival his prowess on the asphalt.

There were groups that trained by themselves and had the dedication to do it, day after day. This was HM2 Chris Parchmon, HM2 [Redacted], and HM3 Ho Vo. They quietly did their thing and did it well.

Back to the prison gym however; it was one of those distinct memories that impressed me as much then as it still does today. We even made an article about it for the *Whiskey Ration.* It was never too hot for them, and they always found the time to get their lifts in. Unfortunately, not everyone will be able to be mentioned by name for their efforts in trying to get in shape, but we did the most we could with what we had. I'm proud of the ingenuity of Whiskey Rotation and will forever tip my hat to them.

5 May 2020
Day 78

It has occurred to me that not only was it Cinco de Mayo yesterday, but also Taco Tuesday. There was a reason I went to get lunch today, and to my chagrin there was no Mexican food served. Lunch was very underwhelming.

Had a majorly good day today, which is more funny than bad, but I had a Navy correspondence question. The question was when writing Lieutenant Junior Grade is the JG capitalized or lowercase? Clearly not a pressing question for anyone. I'd been awake since 0230, and the DFA, Director for Administration, came back from a run around 0400. At 0500 I left the "Coffee Mess" room where I was working and returned to my room. Be reminded that yesterday at 0430 Senior Chief Wink was jaw-jacking with me in the Coffee Mess. When I had the urge for my question, I figured everyone would be awake by now. DFA wasn't in his room, so I went down the line to Senior's place. Well, when he opened the door, he was clearly not awake yet. It was then I looked at my watch and realized I was asking him this stupid question at 0600! Luckily for me he was a good sport about it.

All my articles are finished for Issue #2. Now it's just managing HM3 Writer and getting the last remaining article. Not sure why the diversity article is taking so long. Either way, it felt good to get it all wrapped up. We will see how much is undone during the edit phase.

Postscript: It was mentioned before, but I really do not like revising my own work. I do however recognize that it is a necessary evil, but because I wanted no part in the editing phase of the newsletter, why would I talk negatively about it. It would be more meaningful if I was invested in the complete process, and that was a sign of my immaturity for not appreciating the bigger picture. The newsletter was a document that spread far and wide throughout the Navy, Department of Defense, and into the screens of our parent commands and families. At the time I did not appreciate or understand the situation.

6 May 2020
Day 79

Normally when I write in my journal, I put some thought into what I have to say before there is a pen put to paper. Today that doesn't seem to be the case. Unlike yesterday I was able to sleep enough during the day, and that's good because from the little bit I did experience it was hot. Like, hotter than I was used to.

One thing out of the ordinary today was it was my day to help clean the bathrooms. Too bad I couldn't say it was a high honor, but to be fair it was thirty minutes at most out of my way.

I also watched two guilty favorite movies today, *National Lampoon's: Van Wilder* (2002) and *Ace Ventura: Pet Detective* (1994). With the former, it brought me back to high school and college. Ryan Reynolds has aged well. With the latter, it brought me back to my childhood and reminded me just how many lines and mannerisms my brother Dylan and I ripped from that film. Watching them side-by-side forced me to note how I enjoy films about a character in a league of their own, kept afloat by their own brand of confidence.

Two people on separate occasions over the course of the day saw my notebook and complimented me on my penmanship. That, of course, made me feel good.

Went out again with LT Byrd, and I just noticed how bad the writing was. I can do better. Anyway, a CrossFit Conex box came in. They had a hex-bar, and we did some farmer carries. Somehow, I'm only a little sore and that is an improvement.

Postscript: We are now clearly in a holding pattern at cruising altitude in Qatar. There is so much routine that it is hard to describe what to write about without one entry sounding like a carbon-copy of the day before. Looking back at it I wish I had taken more pictures or kept a record of more things like the temperature or written more details about things no one else would think about at the time, but maybe someone would find it important later, like a historian.

8 May 2020
Day 80 & 81

For some reason it has finally struck me that it's May. That's good and I'm a bit sad. It feels like we've covered so much ground, but in reality, we haven't done squat. Still over 80 days away from home.

Saori thinks the boys, especially Josiah, are acting out in a way that projects their sadness. He throws things in his temper tantrums, hits Saori, and is starting to say he doesn't like this or that. I personally think he's acting out because he can, but then again that's actually what I hope is happening. It's very painful to think about my boy being sad and depressed while his papa is away for work. One day I hope he'll understand, and I hope to one day make it up to him.

I was today-years old when I learned that Military Spouse Appreciation Day is the Friday before Mother's Day every year. In years past, this was something to mock and disregard. Except this year it's a bit different for obvious reasons, and I really do appreciate my spouse in this military life. Saori eats more crap than she probably bargained for when we started out. Like Josiah, I hope to be able to make it up to her one day, because she deserves it.

So, I've been working out with LT Byrd nearly every day. I feel skinnier, but no one has mentioned anything about my appearance yet. To be fair it's only been nine days since we started. The primary/initial soreness and pain is gone. I can PT longer and the aches are more welcome. It's no longer the crippling suffering from months of neglect. Each day I try to wake up sore enough that I can stretch it out before the next workout. I'm only eating two meals a day but throwing in enough snacks to bust the fasting cycle. LT Byrd did say that people have told him it looks like I'm losing weight, but not to me. I think he's just being nice. What I'm doing is waiting for my shorts to not fit anymore. It'll be one fine day when I don't have to wear XXL.

We are in crunch time with *The Whiskey Ration Newsletter*. Only two more days until we have to route it through the Chain of Command. There is plenty to improve on from my perspective. Hopefully I am my own worst critic. Yesterday I used the four magic words, "What do you think?" to LCDR Fitzgerald. Interesting consequence, she hasn't said anything about it but the deputy PAO, LT Simon Prado, did. As I hoped for, I was the harsher critic, and his guidance did not end the entire project.

I'm trying to read more and put down the phone even more than trying to read. It doesn't always work, but I feel much more productive with a made bed, door open, me sitting in my chair with either my Chromebook or a book in my lap. I know it sounds silly, but it reminds me of being in the UW-Green Bay dorms again. I wish I tried to be more creative at a younger age when failure was less consequential and I had less to lose.

Postscript: Whenever I talk about it being a certain day or month, I feel like Nick Carraway from The Great Gatsby *remembering that the day was actually his birthday. Of course, it was May! I had written specifically about it a couple of times previously. Maybe not a lot of thinking was going on, we were pushing at a low enough tempo to just get through the time in Qatar. I really am a sucker for nostalgia because that line about being in the UW-Green Bay dorms doesn't tell the whole story. I never wanted to miss any action, so I would keep my door open, always inviting guests should they choose to visit. It ended up messing up my sleep pattern and I had to see the campus nurse about it. It was the beginning of my bouts of insomnia because it was hard for me to turn off my mind.*

9 May 2020
Day 82

It's another beautiful night here in Qatar. I think I have written every journal entry while in country in the dead of night at this picnic table that sits outside the barracks. This journaling project is something I'm beginning to become proud of because of its longevity.

I just hope my roommate in KAF doesn't mind. That's right, the room list came out yesterday and I played myself by suspending my own expectations. There is no change in who I will be living with, HM2 Terrell. I don't even know his first name by memory yet. It could definitely be worse, but I just don't know the guy. I played myself because for a moment I thought my luck in having my own room would continue. PS2 Robert Krombach, the only Second Class, has his own room. Good for him. What should be interesting is all three enlisted girls are E-4 and below, and two are E-3s. They all get their own rooms. It shouldn't be a thing, nor should it matter, and as long as I don't think too much about it, I won't work myself into a tizzy. At least I'm on the first floor.

Started really getting into the ten-part Michael Jordan documentary *The Last Dance.* If I switch my VPN to Germany, I can watch it on Netflix. I have to download each episode however because streaming quality is not the greatest, but it's free.

Only 200 pages to go in my Laura Ingalls Wilder book. Tomorrow I do another PT test with LT Byrd; good times. Can't wait to get my haircut. I'm feeling like a slummy hippie. I can smell myself.

Postscript: The jockeying for rooms was just another thing we did as an enlisted force to keep ourselves entertained. We have this thing in the military called RHIP, or Rank Has Its Privileges. It usually means that the higher the rank, the easier life gets, and the more perks come your way. Whiskey did a decent job in forgetting about this from time to time, and it shows up later.

10 May 2020
Day 83

I wish there was more today about this day besides Happy Mother's Day. I did my due diligence and called the two mothers in my life. Saori had me talk to Josiah while she ran into the store for some things. We tried to talk, but we just showed each other our stuff instead. He was jazzed about the fireworks he got. I'm happy that he thought highly enough of me to show and tell.

I also cut about 15 minutes off my workout time with LT Byrd. Somewhere along the way, my own stopwatch must have bumped my wrist and showed a time of 17:45. Remember last week my time was 44:14? We took LT's estimate of 30 minutes, but it felt so much better than last week. I also weighed myself today. It's a sign of improvement when you don't send the scale into error. My number today was 295. I'll need to divide by 2.2 in order to get the kilograms.

One thing I've been really feeling lately is the pangs of loneliness. The more I think about it, the more I'm not going to mind having a roommate. Oh! I started to send out my mailing address to everyone. I figured it was time. I won't be expecting much from Japan until the MPS (Military Postal Service) is back to being free. Saori will still pay the postage, but she's special and different and loves me the most.

Newsletter is now routed to the Chain of Command. It has to get through a lot of folks, but hopefully will quickly.

Postscript: To be clear, Saori did not infringe on Japanese norms when she left a five-year-old in the car alone while she ran into the store. Sure, I was "watching" my own child, but I was in Afghanistan. Would have needed to pull some serious Liam Neeson Taken *if things had gone sideways. It's Japan though, so nothing happened. Working through the language divide between my children and I has always been something that made me a little sad about being an international parent, but one day I'll either learn enough Japanese or they will understand enough English to have a normal age-appropriate conversation.*

11 May 2020
Day 84

Just like that, this nightmare is over. Today we received word that we're shipping out tomorrow. The buses are scheduled to pick us up at 0600 and the flight, on a C-17, should be at noon.

No punches are pulled when I try to describe how much this place sucked. For the last supper, we waited in line for 49 minutes to get food. That's how dense the ghetto "Q-Town" has now become.

I know I underscored how isolated and lonely I feel about being in my own room. There is no joy being me, and my paranoid, conspiracy-theory-riddled mind is starting to collect evidence of ostracization. No one would come to my room to get Tide Pods. They'd go to the next building. That's one stupid example. I'm looking forward to being roomed with someone because so far, I'm not having a good time on deployment.

Created a baby name bracket to help friends and family pass the time and for my own entertainment. I even seeded the 42 names. May the best man win, haha. Of course, the "fan vote" will account for 0.0001% in the final decision between Saori and I.

PAO mentioned at 0830 that there were problems with Issue #2. I asked for a 1000 meeting. She said it was perfect. At 1000 she said she needed to take a shower but will be fast. At 1130 she said she was tied up with something else. At noon I walked past the Coffee Mess and she's playing cards. As upset as I am, I know I did my due diligence despite this habitual issue of flaking on agreed upon times.

Postscript: That name bracket was made purely to entertain myself and to give some of the guys a laugh. I was dead set on naming baby #3 Tatanka, but it was quickly voted down in the subcommittee. Saori, not familiar with the NCAA Tournament, did not give my quirky idea much attention.

Part II:
Arrival

14 May 2020
Day 85, 86 & 87

It has been a whirlwind seventy-two hours. Finally! Whiskey has made its final destination. There are so many observations and changes compared to what we are used to; it's just been a lot. Like any story worth its salt, we will begin at the start, or is that the other way around?

Leaving Qatar was relatively easy if you didn't mind the hurry-up and waiting. In that case, we didn't leave the quarantine ghetto, or "Q-Town" until 0600, but we didn't fly until 1300. Lots of checkpoints here and there.

What I did do that was most noteworthy was eat some locally made hummus. I guess it's like eating a cheese curd if you're in Wisconsin. When you're in Rome, one eats as the Romans do. It was delicious and it made me think I could make my own with the boys after I got back, especially after CDR Phil Self mentioned how easy it was to make.

Before landing in Kandahar, we had to stop at Dwyer base. I think it's Camp Dwyer. We had to pick up a truck, and not a common pickup truck either. We flew in a C-17 like the one I flew from Singapore to Yokota, Japan, in 2017. It was fun to see everyone else's face of awe and wonder because they are so big inside.

It was a three-hour flight to Dwyer, and another 45 minutes to Kandahar. When we got off the plane, we were screened for COVID, again. We had one person pop positive and that caused a little delay. Before we could even leave the final hangar, we waited there for another three hours. It wasn't until midnight we found our beds.

That wasn't before walking to the hospital then getting a bus ride to billeting for our room key. We went to the hospital for initial badges, weapon ammunition, and laundry bags. We were all very tired, but we changed roommates anyway before going to bed.

My roommate is now HM2 Justin Drumheller. So far, I made the right call. He talks to his wife at all hours, which is cute because they're expecting their first child in October.

The only two complaints I have for my room itself is my desk chair is whack, it sits too high so my legs can't sit nicely underneath. My second gripe is the clothes wardrobe is too small. Thank goodness for these plastic drawers my sponsor left for me. For the most part, everything fits.

My desk is lined with books ranging from what I mailed from California to my screenwriting books. One surprise I did discover was how buggy it is on base, or in this area. In Qatar it was essentially void of everything except heat. There are more trees than I was expecting, too. One of the fastest and most assured ways to increase troop morale is to have not only good food, but enough food. Our galley, or in Army lingo, DFAC, here is the best. Food is always plentiful, good hours of operation, it tastes good, and it could easily get me in trouble if I don't quickly discipline myself.

I have yet to set foot in the pharmacy. Not only will there be plenty of time for that, but I was shadowing clinic duty yesterday. I had to go get the food and deliver to the clinic, drop-off and pick up laundry, and deliver water to the depots around the building. It took all day, but at least it wasn't hard or overnight.

When I got home, I was gassed. Turned on my Sapphire internet brick and HM1 Wilson messaged me at 1625, "Hey, if you're not actively doing something on duty swing by the pharmacy and wait for me." I saw and replied from my room at 1755, "So I'm going with the Sapphire for now, which of course I only keep in my room. Just saw this message. Once I burn the 15GB, I will reexamine internet provider." Then I turned my phone off, went to dinner, and then the self-service laundry. When I turned my phone on, I got this from HM1 that he sent at 1940, "HM2, I asked you to come by, right? Are you blowing me off? I see your response, but I haven't seen you." This prompted me to immediately call him at 2211. He answered and said we'd talk about it in the morning. I'm very confused but will get to the bottom of that then.

Finally got a haircut today. Shaved clean off. Barber got a nice tip for using rubbing alcohol on my scalp. In essence, I have to get used to working again. I've gotten used to doing only what I wanted to do and therefore have gotten soft. Really thankful for the kompo Saori mailed.

Postscript: Kompo is essentially Chinese medicine. It's granular and tastes awful. There are different kinds that claim to work different cures, but the kind Saori mailed me was supposedly for belly fat. What it really does is clear out your digestive tract. Think fiber on steroids. I remember a lot going on when we first arrived in Kandahar and wondering how I was going to make it all fit in my journal. There was a lot of shuffling to this location or another. Because our trip was delayed by about six weeks, our preceding rotation, Victor, was more than ready to hand over the baton. They were very thorough and prepped to change over command. Overall, it was a lot of information in not a lot of time.

15 May 2020
Day 88

Well, at least we know what that was all about. We have a lounge in the hospital. It has tables, chairs, and couches. Yesterday, during lunch hours, I napped on the couch. Apparently Senior Chief Wink didn't appreciate it and let HM1 Wilson know how he felt. That's why he wanted to see me. Compound that with "blowing him off" and I had the choice of either having a written counseling or work out with him. Needless to say, I chose the latter and for almost an hour he ran me ragged. I know he has the best of intentions but did that hurt! Afterwards we went to the galley together.

At 1400 I had a meeting with the training team for turnover. It doesn't seem like too much to do and a high ceiling if we want to go above and beyond. I'm on the fence if this is the job where I want to hang my hat. HM2 Jesse John was also at the meeting, and he mentioned something to the effect that the transition with the Army will start to begin as early as July. I don't quite know how to handle that rumor. For a guy who requested to extend, that's a nice thought about now.

I'm straight up not having a good time so far. It's nice to finally get to sit at my desk and write a little. I'm caught up with my hardcopy journaling. Now it's all about getting qualified, competent, and most importantly stepping into a consistent battle plan.

I officially hate the Sapphire.

Postscript: The Sapphire was a mobile Wi-Fi brick you could subscribe to and receive internet access anywhere. It was on loan from HM2 Brandon Wydra who was part of Uniform Rotation. The problem was it ate through cash while delivering suspect Wi-Fi. By this time the internet infrastructure in Kandahar was well formed and the Sapphire's utility was antiquated. While I was on duty, I napped in the lounge, and this was not a good look while so much turnover was happening, especially from a Second Class. The irony is that a HN later in the deployment did the same thing, and it was celebrated in the newsletter. Perception is everything I suppose. It did not take long, like the second day, before rumors started swirling about the Hospital's fate. Rumor management was a fun game to play, and you had to really trust your sources.

16 May 2020
Day 89

This will be a day that'll be very hard to forget. It was my first 24-hour shift in the pharmacy, and there was plenty to discuss.

First, three ANA (Afghan National Army) men were flown in. There was a command-wide recall, and you could tell everyone was getting amped up. One man died on the Emergency Room table, but not before the doctors cracked his chest open and massaged his dead heart to pump again. Two other men are now in the Intensive Care Unit (ICU).

For the man that departed, we lined the hall and saluted as he was wheeled to the morgue. His body in a bag with the Afghan flag draped on the top.

There is a huge learning curve here and I wish I could write it all, but the most important observation is I need to get in my repetitions. Get the muscle memory down and hopefully the rest will follow.

I didn't go outside once today, there was too much to do, but I did the seabag drag with all my flack gear. That was heavy, and hopefully I don't need to move it for a long time. I'll need it to protect myself when we screen casualties from outside.

Finally logged into my work Outlook account. There were 762 emails waiting for me since leaving Japan.

The biggest news, like all before wasn't enough, is I was asked again if I wanted to extend until May 2021. I immediately tried to call HMCM Lorenzo Branch. It was too late at night, but the message was passed. I don't know what I must do to be worthy of being a First Class. I have nowhere else to go.

Postscript: This was a real intense day, and we had just started our tour. Although I did little to personally be involved with direct patient care, the Victor Rotation guys were, and when they were finished, one of them had to have a moment to go outside and smoke a cigarette. Ancillary services such as laboratory, radiology, physical therapy, and pharmacy had the responsibility of taking casualties off the ambulances, screening them to ensure they were safe to enter the hospital, and transporting them to the gurneys inside the Emergency Room. They also saw up close what the casualty looked like before anyone else. It could be overwhelming. It was a humbling experience lining up along the hallways as this protector of freedom was taken to the decedent affairs building. Reminded me that this was now real.

19 March 2020
Card From My Parents

Hi Cal,

Our stay-ca is officially underway. We will be taking small day trips as we have a painter coming over. Today, meat market, Dubuque Iowa riverboat, and anything else on our way that's open. Not gonna lie, this and the state of our country has me a little shooken up. Love you #1 son - Mom

Son,

What you are doing for you and your family's future is very much commendable. You are a good man. Keep on making us proud. Love, Dad

27 March 2020
Card From Saori

Husband,

Hope you have arrived in Afghanistan safe and sound, and you are ready for your new adventure. Things are so different here without you and we miss you lots. The Wisconsin flag you put up on the kids' room ceiling is now hanging from one corner, and I really don't know how to fix it without risking the baby and myself. It's so cute to see Josiah put my phone beside his bed, expecting your phone call while I'm reading to them every night. I didn't tell you this sooner because I didn't want you to give up on your gym time in the mornings. We try to support you as much as possible, so please always get your spirit up and do your things. We love you and always wish for your safety and success! Be safe, only 6 more months to go. F&E, Wife

17 May 2020
Day 90

Holy cow, it has actually been 90 days since leaving Japan. I doubt Josiah can even count that high.

From my actions today it may even be more than originally planned. I accepted the request to extend to May 2021 should my command approve it. I have yet to hear from Master Chief Branch, but the question will certainly be put on his desk soon enough.

Today was a peculiar day. I slept well enough; I had an exchange of messages with HM2 Mario Torres before falling asleep. In the morning I called Saori to tell her I might have to extend. To my surprise she was already anticipating it. The details could be saved for another time.

I spend every day in the pharmacy to get as much training and experience as I can before I'm independent. I didn't leave work until 1400 today, and I was ready to leave by that time. When I got home, I became a lazy piece of crap except that I wrote three letters to Grandma Mongin, a card to the boys, and one to my parents.

My new notebook is college-ruled so I left my letters to only one page each. This is very different from my typical three pages per letter. I think that is because I'm duplicating so much information to so many people it does get tiring saying the same things over. Plus, I try to limit my pages to people who I know don't save their letters. My stomach has been messing with me all evening, so I didn't work out. I did clean around my room though to help declutter my mind.

LETTERS FROM HOME

There has been a lot of mention of letters and page-count to this point, and it's as good a time as any to take a dive into what the context behind all that means. It began when I was a tender youth and my family moved from Wisconsin to Nashville. The year was 1997 before the explosion of the Internet. It certainly existed, but its common access was not yet popular, and definitely not popular enough for middle class children to readily use. This was also a time before widespread cellphones and long-distance phone calls were still a thing. Yes, I lived in a time where the yellow pages still meant a thick book the telephone company would deliver to our home once a year.

If you wanted to keep in touch with friends, teachers, or family, we had to write letters. Once a week, in order to keep me and my siblings busy, my mother would make us write letters. I enjoyed doing it, and always appreciated when a letter was returned. To show my appreciation, I kept every letter. This became a habit and since 1997 I have saved every letter ever sent to me. After joining the Navy and moving to Virginia, I took my collection and cataloged them according to date into sleeves of plastic and put them into big binders.

Although it will be said more so later in these pages, writing was something therapeutic to me. I tend to write more when I get in melancholy moods and it does a good job bringing me back to higher spirits. I take writing very seriously, from the pens I use, to the paper I write on, to the style of penmanship. Family lore says that my grandmother has the best penmanship in the family, and whether that is true or not, it remains fact within the Mongin-side of the family.

After my collection had been built up enough, I began to joke that my biographer one day will want to read these primary documents to get a better sense of my life while they build a library that will one day bear my name. To that end, I never wanted to "put in the work" of a lengthy epistle if I knew it would find its way to the trash. For lack of a better word, I find it disrespectful. Finding someone who will take the time to care with their handwriting and say intimate things to you is a gift I believe should be cherished. I typically believed that a three-page letter said enough while not keeping the reader too long. As I increased my number of letters to the array of friends and family while on deployment, the romanticism of writing became mildly burdensome, so I cut back on the page count and hoped that a letter from Afghanistan would be special enough.

Whether anyone keeps my letters or not is a job for my biographer to find out, not me. I am too self-conscious to find out for myself in case they tell me something I would rather not hear. It does not stop me from inking notes when I am thinking about someone though. People sometimes look at me a little sideways when I share with them that one of my hobbies is writing letters. When I'm alone, in my office, and all is quiet about the house, yes, I like to let someone know that they are special enough to me to rate more than an email about the happenings of my life.

Letters are very special to me, and the written word is a precious gift. A typed letter is excused if the sender has awful penmanship, and an email is fine because time was still taken, but it's not the same as fully utilizing the United States Postal Service.

23 May 2020
Day 91, 92, 93, 94, 95 & 96

Clearly there is much to account for. Although there is a lot to discuss, there was also a lot to process and try to understand. Six days from the last entry is in fact inexcusable, but it's not like I've been slumming it either.

I'm back in the workforce and it feels both awesome and exhausting. Of course, I won't go through day by day, but tackle the broad strokes and my feelings or observations of them.

Yesterday was the official change of command when our CO took over. Due to COVID precautions, only senior officers and leadership were permitted to attend. The luncheon afterward was incredible. I'm still thinking about the artistry and time that went into carving and baking and presenting everything. The cake had to be four feet long.

Although Victor Rotation is no longer in charge, they still aren't gone. A flight out of KAF is technically not on the books for them, yet. This means habitual loitering around the hospital like they literally have nothing better to do. It has become a little stressful working beneath them. Granted, I learned a lot about being an impatient pharmacy technician.

My crash course was primarily spread over two 24-hour shifts. I was trained under HM2 (FMF) "Jeremiah". Nice guy out of Lemoore, California. I have been working at the hospital every day trying to learn as much as I could.

Last night was my crucible; my first 24-hour shift by myself. It forced me to stay awake until 0200 trying to figure out the way to do certain procedures. I knew the answers were somewhere I could read on the computer, but I had to go look for it. No doubt in three months it's going to be nothing out of the ordinary to do what I did. At the time, last night, it wasn't traumatic, but it got me excited.

My low-key fear is I will be expected to work every day while the other techs are nowhere to be found on their admin day off. Not sure how LCDR Deguzman does it; he's at work every day. He's also paid the most and doesn't spend the night. Time will tell on these worries.

So far, I still like my roommate, HM2 (SW/AW) Justin Drumheller. He's a lot more relaxed than me and listens well when I complain. He hardly snores and is mindful about using the phone. He's interesting in the sense that he volunteered to extend, but also volunteered to go home early. As of now, there is no change in pharmacy personnel.

Master Chief Branch personally called to say they, Sasebo, could not support me extending. His reasoning was a little off, citing manning with Yani Lopez. At least I have an answer now and can call it a prayer answered in the sense that there is resolution.

Yes, I miss Sasebo. I call it the Shire of my world. Of course, I miss my kids. I can feel my eyes well up with allergies every time I see them. What I really like is when Saori shares with me little stories about them saying how much they miss me too. I don't always get that impression when I'm on the phone with them. A good example though is when Josiah was riding his bike. He could tell Saori was on her phone. Apparently, he said in Japanese not to take a picture, but to call Papa instead. That makes me ache, but it also adds to the romanticism of what a deployment is.

Besides the mail that was waiting for me when I showed up, there was a charming letter from Grandma Judy and a care package from Saori. The letter had two pictures printed on it from '94 and '95. She added a little note, and it definitely raised the morale. Mail is delivered only twice a week here, Monday and Fridays. That takes a little adjusting, but it is a manageable problem.

Issue #2 of *The Whiskey Ration Newsletter* has been published. Although I'm happier with it than Issue #1, there is still room to work. Like Johnny Depp, I don't actually read the final product. In my mind, the end goal or product is what I submitted on the 10th of each month. What edits or revisions that are made after that are not my problem. Probably sounds all sorts of bad, but it is my process to let go and not take it so personally.

Each day I come home exhausted. As much as I would like to blame working out, I feel the main reason is mental distress. Learning inpatient pharmacy has not been fun, and the first couple of days I really struggled. So much so that they were thinking of putting me on days while the First Classes switched days and consequently take overnight shifts too. That would have been embarrassing to me and hardship on them. Luckily, I have been able to pull my act together, and at the eleventh hour I proved competent enough to stand by myself. All of this just adds to my growing frustrations and doubts.

My thoughts have been so down, I wrote a stream of consciousness email to Master Chief Greg Fall. By the time I checked my email the next day he had replied in full. Anything he says is like a screenplay written by the Coen brothers to John Goodman. So yes, what he had to say helped put some things into perspective, and I'll forever be thankful to him for everything he has helped me through. He once told me that there were enough Greg's in the world, but when our third child is born, there will be at least one more, even if it's just a middle name.

The food here remains awesome. Luckily for me I have discovered the salad bar line. Most meals I have are mostly salad or items from that line. Not everything though. I'll save a little compartment for protein and I'm still learning to kick the habit of starches. When the potatoes are real, I get irrationally excited. One guilty pleasure is the yogurt parfait they have. I think once I master the art of portion control, the real progress will start to be seen. Until then, mostly vegetables with my meals. Oh! Every Friday is steak and crab leg night.

Luckily for me, I now have a locker at the hospital. Although it's in the Emergency Department, it's close to the showers and there isn't too much traffic in and out. One thing I will need to get is another hook for my towel to hang outside my door. If I'm being extra greedy, a scale close to the locker would be ideal.

The bed for overnight duty is probably more comfortable than my bed in the barracks. I am not a fan of my desk though, but I am thankful I at least have one. I acquired a different chair to supplement the broken one from LT Byrd. It is either too high, or I'm too tall. Either way, my legs don't fit underneath. Not exactly what one might call ergonomically inclined.

I started to memorize the Rudyard Kipling poem "If." For no other reason than to please and entertain myself. There isn't that much more to expand on that until it's complete.

So far, I feel quite misled about the level of downtime we have here. I'm looking at all my books in front of me, and I don't know when I'll ever get to them all. Again, it'd really help if I could just put down the damn phone. I'm super behind on my letters, creative writing, and reading. That doesn't include learning Japanese. I think that was one reason why I wanted to extend, to find more time to get to those kinds of projects. By writing that, I recognize how stupid that sounds.

Maybe I really want to know what it's like to suffer. I'm so blessed and, throughout this entry in particular, lucky to have so many goals and things in my life. I know that I have zero concept of what a truly bad day is. Maybe I want to know what another sacrifice feels/looks like compared to my peers, especially my civilian counterparts. I'm beginning to feel more and more that I have reached my terminal paygrade. That thought is absolutely terrifying. It was the crux of my conversation with Master Chief Fall. Job security is an ever-increasing value I have.

One more thing, my Manitowoc Minute Sconnie flag is now here.

Postscript: Clearly, I had a lot going on in my mind. I was so desperate to use this deployment as a last stand to show my worthiness for promotion that it might have clouded other things, like enjoying the experience. That was something I always struggled with because people enjoying the moment are generally not moving, and if you're not moving upward, then what are you doing with your time? Even though I don't know what my peak will be, I know it's not here, and that's why I'm constantly driven to not be where I am. It kills my mother to read these types of thoughts, and I understand her position, but there is always an itch I can't scratch.

24 May 2020
Day 97

Incredible to think that I am almost done with writing in this journal. I have two more volumes on standby for when that day comes.

Keepin' 'er movin', I discovered a new full body workout, tire flipping. Freddie, the supply warehouse contractor, has been very supportive and this day we bumped it up a notch. Normally I only knock out pushups each time I visit the supply guys, and there are three of them: Sean, Eugene and Freddie. Long story short, I was absolutely gassed by the end of my exercise, but encouraged to do it tomorrow, and the next day, etc.

Watched *JoJo Rabbit* (2019) with Drumheller today. He's always making German jokes, he's from Pennsylvania, and I really enjoy the movie craftsmanship. He liked it too.

Something happened today, I had my first day off from work. It was everything I thought it would be. Caught up on my journaling, took a nap, going to write a letter or two, and thinking about Issue #3 of the newsletter. Called my mom too, and we talked for like 50 minutes. It was the first time in two weeks we talked.

We now have a power converter, which will support keeping our fridge both on and cold. My water intake had jumped up considerably. Today reached 100 degrees and it felt like it.

Also had ice-cream on the boardwalk. Not worth it.

Postscript: Kandahar used to be a booming base. Although I could never confirm it, rumor has it that there used to be a TGI Fridays restaurant. In the middle of the base was the boardwalk, a covered walkway that had little shoppettes, and vendors around its fringes. Inside of the boardwalk was the athletic field, which held a soccer pitch, 400m track, and outdoor gym. In the winter years ago when the Canadians had a larger presence on the base, they would fill the outdoor gym area and play hockey on it. COVID took all that away. By the time Whiskey Rotation showed up, it was a shell of itself. By the time we left, it was even more desolate, and I think this paired with the eventual shutdown of the base.

25 May 2020
Day 98

Holy cow am I tired. It is my duty day and, I look at my watch, it is 2358. I wish I could say I was reading my book or something for me, but it was all for the glory of the pharmacy tonight. Although it certainly wasn't as stressful as my last duty day, it remained meticulous. I guess I'd rather have it that way than being absent-minded.

I worked out today. During my workout I knocked out 60 pushups and I was surprised how easy it felt. It gave me hope I could do 40 more with the warehouse guys later in the day. How mad I got when they told me what pushups I do outside don't count. What matters is what I do in front of them, and as far as they were concerned, I did zero for the day. I told them it was fertilizer and went ahead and did five sets of 20 throughout the day. Needless to say, I was more sore than I wanted to be, but I'm happy I did it.

Again, I feel like I failed at the spoon discipline aspect. I'm starting to miss breakfast again and drink lots of water instead. Oh, I pooped I think four times today, which is of course very weird for me. It wasn't diarrhea either. Maybe all the fiber? I'm going to really enjoy my shower tonight.

Wrote to HN Pham.

Postscript: Behind the hospital was the Swole 3 gym. Not sure where the "3" came in, but to get swole is a contemporary term meaning to get big and feel the pump. Swole 3 was under tactical tarps but completely outside. It consisted of a squat rack, bench press, incline press, pullup bar, dumb bell set, and an exercise bike. Maybe some more stuff, but that was essentially it. Every other rotation was able to enjoy the huge indoor gym in the building next to the barracks. COVID closed that down; we never saw it open. Next to Swole 3 was a basketball court and tires for flipping. What I coined as "Freddie Tire Flips" consisted of flipping the tire, hopping in and out to the other side, hopping back to the original start point, and flipping the tire again to complete one set.

27 May 2020
Day 99 & 100

Happy 100th day anniversary. Is this a happy day? It certainly isn't, and in order to leave some perspective we are not even halfway through what it could be if we come home in mid-October, like what Brandon Wydra did.

Speaking of, I found his radiology book that he left when he was part of Uniform Rotation. That is kind of cool that it was still here, but on the other hand there was only one rotation of separation. I should mail it back to him with my latest copy of *Family Handyman* magazine.

Yesterday was a little interesting in the sense that I handled my post-duty "admin" day way better than last time. A shower goes a long way, and I'm thankful that there's plentiful enough running water for that to happen. I was tanked, though, by 1130 when released, so I went home and took a nap. After waking up, it was a quick phone call home and then back to the hospital for the Diversity Committee meeting to plan for Pride Month in June.

The most exciting part of yesterday was preparing all the meds for three Afghan nationals that have been inpatients since we arrived. We thought the plane was leaving like now, so it was quite the production. Technically I wasn't ordered or asked to help, but I knew about the rush, so I stepped inside the Thunderdome anyway. It is HM1 Wilson's duty day, but it really showed how far he has transitioned from technician to Chief in training. Multiple times he has expressed gratitude for me stepping up and in. I shared with him that this was the way, and I need him to be the best HM1 he can be to help me the most as a HM2. In order for that to happen, I need to do my part and keep him from getting lost in the technician sauce if I can help it.

So now it's my day off. I slept until 1000 and it felt amazing. Laid in bed until 1230 when I dropped off my laundry at the self-service 'mat. To my surprise it was only a 9-minute walk. It takes longer to get to the hospital.

It's starting to get hot, real hot. Like an old man, I'm sitting outside writing, protecting my clothes, finding time to write. It's hot though, and I said it again because it was worth mentioning.

Will definitely need to PT tonight at the hospital. Took yesterday completely off, not even pushups.

Oh, the three patients? They ended up leaving at 0400 today. We had that big rush for nothing, which only gives us one patient left in the hospital. Honestly, I try not to think about this patient because I know they're like two years old and it's rumored that if they're released to a local host nation hospital that they will likely die. I'd rather not become too attached; forgive me.

Postscript: There were three pharmacy technicians, and we each covered a certain aspect of the job better than the others. HM1 LaPenna was the best technician, HM1 Wilson was the best administrator, and then there was me who was happy to be there. My natural tendency was to lean towards Wilson's style, but LaPenna was a good example too. Of course, they were both First Classes and had to do both, but they were just better at some things than others. I always admired that, but that's not how it always seemed.

28 May 2020
Day 101

For only having one patient admitted, I am more tired than I ought to be. It was probably from my workout this morning after taking two full days off. No, I didn't PT last night. We were recalled to the hospital in order to assist with helping Victor Rotation get on out of here by doing a seabag drag. There were too many Indians helping out, so I went to the pharmacy to jaw jack with HM1 Michael LaPenna.

We found out that it was an officer who left a loaded gun on a bench for hours. Nothing will happen because she's an officer. Nothing we will ever know about at least.

Back to the original news, Victor Rotation is leaving tonight. Also, 20 staff on Victor earned a Bronze Star. I'm sure the citations were riveting and accurate.

PT was a beast. Of course, I flipped more tires today, but I also took two 25 lb plates and walked up the stairs which led to the roof of the hospital.

I did three sets of three reps (up and down). Yes, I was pretty gassed afterwards. Also, I did 105 pushups today for the supply guys.

Started working on *The Thirsty Camel.* Letters sent to HMCM Branch and LCDR Chris Rock.

Postscript: For everyone in Whiskey Rotation reading this, we know who left the gun out. For everyone wanting me to name drop, in another life I might have, but I can confirm justice was served swiftly and without prejudice. I'm just glad it wasn't me. All those Bronze Stars are still talked about among the Whiskey guys, and there isn't anything we can do about it. I do have a feeling that there was an inflation of personal awards every other rotation, and it just happened that Whiskey brought us back to reality to ensure the further integrity of an End of Tour (EOT) award.

29 May 2020
Day 102

These are interesting times. On one hand, I want to go out and exercise, but on the other, I'm tired and feel I'd be most comfortable in my bed.

I did however write a letter to my friend Robert. The way it's looking, one might think that I write very particular things to certain people. It's not like I'm purposely hiding anything from anyone. In fact, I think it is more knowing your audience. For obvious reasons I don't write about my failures and embarrassment during this deployment to Grandma Mongin, but I will to Robert.

The day started off a little rockier than I would have preferred. The ICU was looking for a medication I didn't know how to exactly make, and I felt incompetent. Overall, it was a learning experience, especially since they didn't end up needing the medication to begin with. I have been picking up on a disturbance in the Force though. My two other pharmacy co-workers are seemingly picking a "fight" with other departments, especially the nurses, and by proxy they are taking it out on me. They are the nurses. Everyone wants as little of a workload, and everyone has an idea how that can happen. I think that is where the budding problem is coming from.

Called home and Josey was already sleeping. Atticus was laying with his mom, and it was so cute to see. I cried.

Postscript: In case it was not obvious, here's a little backstory on my friend Robert. Before I left, he was considered my best friend in Sasebo. He had this thing where he always talked about his last command in Sigonella, Italy, but never about anywhere else. I knew that he was once "greenside," serving with Marines, and was deployed before, but he never talked about it. He said, "Because I actually did shit," when talking about his deployment history. It's the men and women like Robert that made this project so hard to write. They actually did shit and had to spend time on a couch talking about it with professionals. I had running water, air-conditioning, and my own computer. Our deployments were not the same, and I will never be able to pretend like they were. The fights that the more senior pharmacy techs were picking in my eyes was actually them not being picked on and abused. They worked in real hospitals before; I did not.

31 May 2020
Day 103 & 104

Pretty good day to close out the month. For the last couple of days, I've been listening to Jocko Willinik's podcast. For the most part, I don't like his stuff, or at least what YouTube is recommending to me. I guess I have to separate his "legend" from the fact that he's still a human who laughs, jokes, and has a family.

One thing in reverse order, *The Thirsty Camel* has been leaked/released. It's quickly turning into the worst lie that no one knows who wrote it. We will see tomorrow when hospital leadership walks in. Maybe I'll be grabbed by the neck fat, but first reports from the populus are that it was extremely entertaining. Time will tell I suppose, but I'm so far proud of my work.

I also interviewed LCDR Claudine Bansil for *The Whiskey Ration.* She will be placed in the Sailor in the Spotlight feature along with three other people.

Today is my 24-hour shift. I feel we are definitely starting to cruise now. I was able to see the night crew in the Patient Administration Department (PAD) working on their college classes. Well, I'm not doing college here. There is Navy e-learning to do and eventually Japanese. That will come.

Finally, I finished my Laura Ingalls Wilder biography. The thing I found to be the most interesting was it all circled back to Laura's father and her love for him. In that way it was really touching, but on the other hand, I felt it dragged on and on. The relationship between her and her daughter was examined so closely it was a bit of a turn-off.

Now I'm back to reading Stephen King and *Dr. Sleep*. My mom inscribed a copy for Christmas. King's books are, in my opinion, a quick read. Hopefully I'll finally Facebook less and pick up the book more.

Today wasn't a good workout. To atone for my failure, I did 140 pushups throughout the day with the supply guys. I've been slacking the past few days in the sense that I only am out getting it in the morning of my 24-hour shift. I should be more dedicated to suffering a little more. Sounds crazy, but that's where I'm at. I think my diet is starting to come around. Next step is to record my workouts and look back on my progress. It can only help.

Last night my mom called me. She was with Grandma Mongin. I can't imagine being 93 and ready to die how she is. I think she's being aggressive enough about it with her kids so they start accepting it too.

The Wydra family and Zach Nebus came over to begin landscaping the fire pit. I'm getting jazzed about it. Only wish I could be there.

Postscript: As mentioned before, this book is dedicated to my Grandma Mongin. Her influence and inspiration are referenced all across these pages. She had 10 children, three sets of twins, and a long life. I owe so much to her for how she sees the world. No one is perfect, but she was damn close to it in my eyes. I've gone on to read Jocko's books, and like any piece of literature, you have to pick what is important to the you and use it to assist your own mold of who you are and what you wish to become.

1 June 2020
Day 105

Today *The Thirsty Camel* made its introduction, and it did not disappoint. In fact, it shattered every metric of expectation I could think of. It was overwhelmingly popular. Of course, this makes me feel good. Senior Chief loved it and said as much. But I still have not heard anything from CO or XO. Even my joke about LCDR Fitzgerald went over well and she took it in stride. Without reading it however, my roommate Justin Drumheller threw severe caution and even recommended to cease and desist from further publication. He backtracked when I named some other article headlines, and I know he spoke from a place of love and concern.

The other big news today was I weighed myself, supposedly on a calibrated scale. Since leaving Japan I have lost four pounds. That is it. Of course it has weighed heavily on me. Tonight I had a long meeting with LT Byrd to recalibrate. Together, we have determined that I ingest too much sugar with soda and fruit especially, my portion sizes are too big (I eat with bowls now and not plates), I don't get enough water, and I need to get used to being hungry. There is no substitute; quit being weak-minded. No one can out-train a bad diet and I am no different. Maybe I will try to get more jogging in.

Postscript: That was a pivotal conversation with LT Byrd. More will be written about him, but I tried to stick to his recommended course of action. Drumheller was my own psychotherapist, and I do not believe I would have been able to do half of what I wanted if he wasn't my roommate. I'm a better person for knowing him and without question stood upon his shoulders more than once.

Definitely not a NATO Role 3 MMU publication

The Thirsty Camel

June 2020 **Volume 1, Issue 1**

Special points of interest:

- **If you can't laugh at yourself, you're in for a rude surprise.**
- **King Neptune's team of sea lawyers vetted this article for accuracy and authenticity.**
- **HM1 Wilson did not write this issue (and now he's at least mentioned)**
- **Humor comes from a place of love, important to remember that part.**

Inside this issue:

ICU DH Interview	2
DON and WhatsApp	2
Maui Selected	2
Goat Locker Changing Sails	3
LT Quinn Submitted for Award	3
Deputy PAO guns for top spot	3
Netflix reboots cult classic	4

SEA Doesn't Need Leg Day

Whiskey Rotation's senior enlisted has bragged that leg day is not needed to bury his Sailors.

Senior Chief(FMF) Cam Wink continuously misses leg day, and it is beginning to show for the crew to ridicule him behind his back.

Unfortunately the joke is on the bluejacket enlisted force. With calves smaller than his biceps, the Whiskey "top" can still bury anyone without a second thought.

Each and every day the team is placed upon the back of Senior Chief Wink, but despite all that carrying, the gains are not coming.

Officers bitching or junior Corpsmen crying, it doesn't matter because Senior Wink is there to rub bellies and not give a single damn about himself.

"All he does is put out fires," says one source who wishes to remain anonymous. "If he spent half as much time on himself as he did for the entire Whiskey team maybe he wouldn't look so much like an oddly shaped Dr. Seuss character."

The fact remains that with so much power stored in that little star above his anchor, leg strength is not necessary when it comes to rolling over his subordinates. Lost orders, missing awards and little white lies are just part of the job description.

What is also part of the job is attending boring meetings that no one cares about nor pretends to enjoy. With so many perks to the job, it is no wonder why not more Sailors are Senior Enlisted Advisors.

Maybe we could all take a page from Top's playbook.

Chief Medical Officer for Congress?

Captain Daniel Kahler, the Chief Medical Officer of the rotation that is Whiskey, is allegedly considering a run for the open seat in the House of Representative seat in his home state of California after waking up to realize that the hair which sits upon his head is of congressional quality.

The good Captain has all the stats for a dominating run in the House. he's tall, chiseled jawline and the peppered hair makes him a dominating force to be reckoned with.

The last great California-born politician was Richard Nixon, so the bar isn't set particularly high. No official word is expected to come from the senior Naval Officer's office until after the deployment, but it is speculated that fundraising phone calls have already been made and "temperature" polls ordered.

The Thirsty Camel

Chewing Tobacco Proven to Turn You into a Sexual Tyrannosaurus

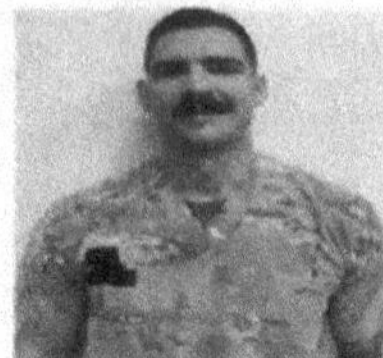

Before

A man who may look like Ron Jeremy.

After

Under normal circumstances, a department head can not be bothered to disclose anything of use. That is why it has been deemed as a high honor for the Thirsty Camel to get insider access to the mind of one of the most brilliant specimens of Whiskey Company, ICU's Dept Head.

In an exclusive interview, it was disclosed that a recent independent study confirmed that chewing tobacco can indeed turn you into a sexual tyrannosaurus. This news is particularly endearing because it seems to be an apt replacement to proper diet and exercise.

ICU's Dept Head also serves as a recon commando medic under the experienced leadership of

Think Jesse Ventura in flick from 1987

ICU Dept Head

Major Arn "Dutch" Anderson. His latest mission was thought to be in the Southeastern Asia jungles, but details are still murky.

When not lifting extraordinary amounts of iron or slicing off a plug of Havana's finest, this ICU Department Head is often seen straight lining copious amounts of southern sweet tea into his veins.

"Becoming a sexual tyrannosaurus is a dangerous game to play," says the DH, "it causes territory wars at KAF and chewing just like me will make a lesser man join the CIA and push pencils for a living." The facts are undisputable.

DON Caps Number of WhatsApp Groups

"There is a fine line between an efficient fighting force and beating a dead horse"

A shockwave is ripping senior Navy leadership to its core after a message was released by SECNAV. In a recent NAVADMIN, it was announced that Commanding Officers must limit the number of WhatsApp groups they subject their Sailors to.

"There is a fine line between an efficient fighting force and beating a dead horse," says part of the message.

This story has been building up for years, and the highest levels of DOD leadership have finally heard the call. One short, balding Senior Chief, "I remember when I could punch out of work and actually relax on deployment. If I heard bombs I knew it was time to head back to the BAS."

Although WhatsApp was created by DON scientists, it has turned into Frankenstein's monster, stealing all joy and privacy from the world's most lethal fighting force.

The message stresses that no more than two WhatsApp groups may be authorized. Any other groups a Sailor must enter is subject to Admiral's Mast under the UCMJ.

Rodriguez Mistaken for Maui, Solicited for Autograph

Whiskey Rotation's HM2(FMF) Jed Rodriguez has been thought to be a fictional Disney character the other day while at the DFAC and asked for an autograph.

A foreign national of undisclosed origins was convinced that he had met Maui from the film "Moana," and would not leave the radiology technician alone until he walked away with either a strand of his hair or an autograph.

HM2 played along as much as he could, signing the admirer's face mask with the inscription, "it's always nice to meet a fan." Afterwards the fan shed a tear of appreciation and left the DFAC without ever getting food .

When dodging the barber, HM2 can be found slinging the iron and designing his next sleeve of tattoos. He's not the demi god we need, but the one we all deserve here at Whiskey.

Not a Disney character voiced by The Rock

"HM2 Rodriguez"

Page 2

Volume 1, Issue 1

KAF Goat Locker Adjusting Priorities

In the geographic area which Afghanistan sits, it is nearly impossible to grow and cultivate Sailors in today's climate. That is why in a recent Chief Petty Officer Association meeting it was decided that Chiefs will now focus their attention to evolving Pokémon instead of their Sailors.

With an emphasis on the Pokémon Go phone application, Chiefs are finding it much more beneficial to their own joy and well-being. Because most "Goats" have children, they can make them happy by growing Pokémon which are exclusive to certain parts of the world. Traditionally, the Afghani species are the hardest and most rare to catch.

Not only are Chiefs doing this for their own families, but they are selling these Pokémon back as fundraisers instead of car washes during initiation season.

One Chief may have said, "these kids just don't listen to humans anymore. They are more interested in learning from Siri and Dr. Google more than 'technical experts' such as Chief Petty Officers."

The bluejacket community is used to getting "fertilized" on by the Goats of the Navy, but their entitled minds and self-pandering mentalities are fighting back stating that Chiefs are no longer mainstream.

Deputy PAO Guns for Top Spot

Whiskey Rotation's second in command to craft public message is itching to get into the pilot's seat. LT Simon Prado allegedly said, "I can't think of any other reason to be on this deployment than to deal with Rastall's bullshit."

The person in question is the prima donna HM2 Cal Rastall, who gave himself the self-proclaimed title of "managing editor" of the monthly publication "Whiskey Ration."

LT Prado believes that there would be no higher joy than to listen to someone bitch and make such a big deal over a monthly periodical which no one actually reads, just looks at the pictures.

"He acts like every issue is going to be submitted for the damn Peabody Award for extraordinary journalism," said a close source, "Between his ears he's Ted Koppel. Hell, he's not even Brian Williams."

Despite what he thinks of himself, Prado knows what he truly is and that's all that matters.

Top Whiskey media whisperer, LCDR Fitzgerald, was not available for comment. She was last seen on her own program sleeping with her weapon under her pillow.

"I can't think of any other reason to be on this deployment than to deal with Rastall's bullshit."

LT Quinn Able to Take Joke, Submitted for Legion of Merit

Some journeys are longer than others, but one thing is certain, everyone loves a good story. No story is more poignant than that of LT Lori Quinn, who was finally able to take a joke at the Spades table. For her actions she is being submitted for the Legion of Merit.

Normally reserved for senior officers under the most austere conditions, LT Quinn was able to finally play along and eat some of the shit she tried to dish out while playing Spades with other enlisted Sailors.

"It's nice to see that she has finally remembered her roots," said a source close to the subject. "LT Quinn wasn't much fun to be around, but now she's okay."

LT Quinn is a former enlisted Sailor and someone forgot that little fact when entering into the Spades Thunder Dome. Her evolution is one to be admired and mimicked and all Bronze Star recipients can now suck it.

POLITICAL CORRECTEDNESS

Whiskey Helps.

When officers start drinking Monsters to be more in touch with the enlisted

Leonardo DiCaprio as Calvin Candy holding a Monster Energy drink asking, "any of you fine gentlemen have a pinch of tobacco?" It's a funny meme, but I can't use it.

Netflix "Twins" Reboot Casting Complete

After an exhaustive effort, the casting for the new "Twins" reboot has been finalized announced Netflix studio heads.

Jackadia Neuman, a Netlix executive stated that "Dr. Gerrid Warner and Edward Howell will be cast to fill the shoes that once belonged to our good friends Arnold Schwarzenegger and Danny DeVito."

The 1988 movie has since turned into a cult classic, on par with Rocky Horror Picture Show and The Big Lebowski. "The studio felt like it was time to see another giant and his vertically inclined sidekick go bombing around the city looking for the next great adventure," Neuman elaborated.

One thing is for certain, Warner and Howell will have on-screen chemistry. After weeks of rooming together in the many shitholes the Navy provided in route to Kandahar, Afghanistan, they have built a form of stamina that is not often seen.

Another studio exec compares the two recast misfits as the next Cheech and Chong, Redford and Newman, or Depp and Bonham-Carter.

Filming is scheduled to begin sometime after their obligation to the service is finished, and after this deployment that is expected to be much sooner than originally anticipated.

Netflix

Arnold and DeVito movie poster here. Because copyright.

4 June 2020
Day 106, 107 & 108

I feel like there is a lot to write about, but it's the type of stuff I need to be on top of otherwise it'll lose its value. What I mean is that there are many flashes of journal-worthy experiences and anecdotes, but like bumping your hip into the counter, the pain and experience quickly get forgotten after it has subsided. In other words, there is nothing systemic going on which is drawn out.

I have noticed my temperament/self-esteem is related to my fatigue. Yesterday I actually jogged on our track. It is a quarter-mile track too. It took me 39 entire minutes to compete three miles. That is a time I can't tell anyone, but do share that as a baseline time establishment, and that part is true. I was tired, but motivated, so I thought it wise to then go to the hospital and go do 24 Freddie Tire Flips. The way it's written in my "Fitness Logbook" is +3, meaning the width of the court plus an additional three flips along the length of the court. One day it'll read "w+l+3…" and so on until I do one complete lap. Either way, this all happened the morning of my 24-hour duty, and I was just wiped out.

HM1 Wilson, who on his day off showed up trying to convince me at 1600, one of the hottest times of day to work out with him, was not received very kindly by me. I appreciate and understand he wants to help, and maybe I was being mentally weak, but he wasn't out there flipping tires at 0600 with me either.

My eating is starting to get straight, I guess. The first night of the "no-plate, just bowl" diet, or LT Byrds's "just get used to going to bed hungry" diet really hurt. It has since tempered off those painful pangs of discomfort. Only using a bowl really helps with the portion sizes, and I enjoy putting salad, beans, veggies, and grilled chicken breasts in my bowl. I drink 1-2 cans of Diet Coke per day too, but in a caloric deficit diet that might be okay. I'm getting plenty of water too. So it's diet, exercise, and sleep.

The third leg of this tripod is what's messing me up. Lately I am finding it hard to "turn my brain off" at night. I'm constantly thinking about something. Generally, it's about writing projects. Either *The Thirsty Camel* or other gigs such as the LGBT ceremony we're to have later this month. I am making a speech and it needs to be no more than five minutes long. I'm excited for the challenge yet very unfamiliar with the material. That's why I'm probably doing this. Looking over the month, I have been writing more than I ever have before. Part of me hopes and expects a dividend to this investment of time and budding talent, but that's just it, budding talent. I might be the "emerging writer" to Whiskey Rotation, but my work might still be crap. It has been a long time since I've been in the company of peers who actually enjoy what I do.

In the world of PAO, I am working on a series which observes the 78th anniversary of the Battle of Midway. Each day I put together a one-page visual presentation. What it's teaching me more than anything is how to better use Microsoft Publisher. It's a neat little program.

Did I ever mention that I'm the Master of Ceremonies for the 122nd Hospital Corpsman Birthday here? Kinda cool, hopefully it might lead to bigger opportunities.

I always thought that June 5 was my graduation day from high school. This paired well with my college graduation date, only 15 years later. Now Facebook is telling me that it is in fact June 4th. Although this might be true, I will continue to say I graduated college 15 years after high school to the day.

Saori picked up the new van today and the boys love the new DVD screen.

Oh! HM2 Foreed Bonsu dropped in. He's at a Role II base about a 30-minute flight away. Cherished moment.

Postscript: Bonsu was a guy I first met in Iwakuni when I was stationed there. Like many people we meet in the military, we remember people based on where they are or where they're going. Admittedly Facebook helps with this a lot. I was always fond of

Bonsu, and it really was a joy to meet up with him so far from where we first met. It was even more neat to see him as the same rank as me, especially since I met him as a HN.

6 June 2020
Day 109 & 110

I want to say that it's been an interesting past couple of days, but it has almost literally been filled with sleeping and work.

From when I last wrote, I did not go to bed. Instead, I wrote a letter to Bandon Wyrda. Because he was previously stationed here in Uniform Rotation, he knows this place, so I can speak to him the most openly about life here. It was a couple of pages long for me to practice my handwriting I suppose.

I honestly thought jogging was going to wire me up, but it did the opposite. I read for a couple hours and then walked over to the hospital where I read some more, but this time I was waiting for my friend HM2 Bonsu who was flying out at 0400. He was surprised to see me, and I think he appreciated the gesture. We said our goodbyes and took a picture that gathered over 130 likes, highly uncommon for a picture of mine. Again, it was so nice to see a familiar face and get to bond with someone. For a suspended moment in time, it was my favorite part of being here. After Bonsu left, I stuck around the hospital and worked on my Midway presentations. That was fine until 0530 when the ICU called for a narcotic order. After that, I helped with the outdoor gym, Swole 3, as it was getting a renovation with space utilization and netting as a cover. That was actually a disorganized mess, so I went to get breakfast then went home.

I wasn't asleep for 2.5 hours until being woken up by my roommate. The Midway presentation, which was sent to PAO for review, was never forwarded to Chief AT despite LCDR Fitzgerald being at work. Chief was getting on my case. As I walked back to the hospital, I was pissed to the highest degree.

Oh, before sleeping, Saori calls me literally crying because of the harassment she was getting from the Sasebo Safety Office clerk. She was so upset, and I don't blame her for not knowing Navy lingo, or being upset at the bureaucracy of something as stupid as a driver's license to drive in Japan when she's a Japanese citizen.

So I stayed at work until about 1600. I called home, but the boys were already sleeping. Instead of taking the 15-minute walk to the new galley, I popped two Benadryl and went to bed at 1730. I woke up a couple of times across the night but fell back asleep until 0600. I felt great.

It's beginning to get hot, real hot. The digital thermometer says 122 degrees Fahrenheit. I took a video of it. Today is refusing to end. It's already 0145 on the 7th. We had two late patients. LCDR Deguzman came back and helped big time. HM1 LaPenna too. Hopefully HM1 Wilson won't expect much from me when he clocks in tomorrow.

Began working on the next *Thirsty Camel.*

Postscript: I hated doing that Midway presentation. It was something that Chief came to me and said it had to be done. To be clear, I agree it is important to recognize our naval history and heritage. On the other hand, it was five straight days of research and trying to put together a visual display I doubted many people actually saw and even less cared about. Since this was a public relations piece, it needed to be vetted through the PAO, but that day was particularly irksome. Miscommunication and missed messages happen all the time. It was a chance for me to grow nonetheless.

8 June 2020
Day 111 & 112

Holy cow do I feel a lot better since taking my shower. It was like a second gust of wind got beneath my wings. Feeling more refreshed, I'm now motivated to write in my journal instead of waiting one more day or even more. I've been thinking lately about starting to transcribe again into Google Docs, and genuinely feel that day is getting closer now that my other writing obligations are winding down. For example, I just completed the second issue of *The Thirsty Camel* today. Unfortunately, it has only been eight days since the last issue was published. There will be no chance to wait more than two more weeks between issues.

In the meantime, I need to get busy with other projects or begin to stockpile issues. I don't know yet how I will handle it. What I do know is that I'm paying a lot of attention deciding what I think is funny. There were entire articles that have been replaced with a completely different premise as a better idea pops into my head. There's a definite game between over-thinking the formula and getting the balance just right.

Last night I called my mom. We spoke close to 45 minutes, and she insisted I forward her a copy of *The Thirsty Camel* Issue #1. Still waiting to hear back from her.

One email I did get a reply to was from Master Chief Greg Fall about stoic leadership. Maybe one day I'll transcribe the email from him since I always seem to forward them anyway to my Padawans saying that "this is what real leadership looks like."

Today we started Operation Cut Fluid Bags in Conex Box. I personally devoted almost three hours of the day to cutting bags of IV fluids which were tainted due to being in a hot Conex box. There are easily over two thousand bags waiting for my attention. Some people helped; most didn't. I'm sure it'll be a nice little memory even without the aid of this journal.

One thing I haven't done is PT or any kind of pushups or exercise in general. Although I do feel bad about that, I also feel as if the days are starting to really fly by.

Final articles for *The Whiskey Ration* are submitted and edited. Might just meet our deadline finally.

Postscript: The transcription onto Google Docs never happened while in Kandahar. I couldn't access my Google account on a government computer, and in order to use my laptop, I would need to disconnect the Wi-Fi from my phone which made it inconvenient. Also, when logged onto the Wi-Fi with my Chromebook (otherwise known as laptop), the language would be really weird, and it just felt like I was being spied on. It didn't work out, and I had to wait until I got back to America for the great transcribing. No one knew how bad COVID was going to be, and the Department of Defense was going to make sure they were prepared. Those IV fluids were a perfect example. Thousands of bags went to waste. They showed up during the Victor Rotation, it was winter, so they put them in the Conex box. Summer came, and they spoiled. Seeing this waste of supplies was too common, but in some regards it was better to be safe than sorry.

DEFINITELY NOT ROLE 3 MMU PUBLICATION

VOL: I ISSUE: II

JUNE DEUX

THE THIRSTY CAMEL

INSIDE THIS ISSUE:

Sailor Chases Record	2
SUPPO's Career	2
KAF Event Rep Selected	2
Combat Pharmacy	3
Halloween Costume	3
Brain Surgeon Problems	3
HM1 Makes Mistake	4
Anchors Away	4

Special points of interest:

- The Thirsty Camel is released whenever the publisher damn well feels like it good and proper.
- HM1 Wilson has been mentioned. End of bullet.
- HM2 Rastall does not endorse any of these articles, and frankly neither should anyone else.
- HN Valdez is only a "lion tamer" in her own mind. Really she's just kitty trafficker of wild animals.
- If you can't laugh at yourself, you're in for a rude surprise.
- King Neptune's team of sea lawyers vetted this publication for accuracy and authenticity.
- Humor comes from a place of love, and fact, important to remember that part.

Arboleda Enrolls in Downey School for Youngsters Who Can't Lift Really Really Good

Rejoice! HM2 Arboleda has finally enrolled in the highly successful Downey School for Youngsters Who Can't Lift Really Really Good (DSYWCLRRG). After seeing the progress and testimony from previous apt pupils, Petty Officer Arboleda is ready to make the plunge.

Previously known as the "Hurt Locker," The DSYWCLRRG was sued back to the Stone Age over copyright infringement. LT Greg Downey, the founder and only faculty of the school, has pulled off the genius move of now mixing two different schools into one.

Meanwhile Arboleda is trying to not get into the weeds with the legal dynamic of a school which makes him want to get swole. Arboleda was previously under the tutelage of HM1 Kubil and HM2 Rodriguez, but it became problematic from an early stage in the process.

Arboleda allegedly suggested that the First Class "didn't smile enough or smoke his flavor of vape." He went on to suggest anyone who is that good at basketball, but is that funny looking belongs in the service of Ringling Bros and not the United States Navy.

The main issue with HM2 Rodriguez was he was too busy shooting all those x-rays in radiology to find the time to get his own pump on, let alone have some novice follow him around the yard.

Trusty sidekick and former padawan LT Taylor has agreed to share LT Downey's off-time and ride the pine while the Good Lieutenant builds up a junior Sailor.

Arboleda does what many won't do so one day he can do what many can't. Investments pay dividends over time. HM2 works hard and it's noticed.

Absolutely ripped from the X-Men Xavier House for Youngsters, but it's a homage to a different film.

The Downey School for Youngsters Who Can't Lift Really Really Good.

LSS: Proposal to Move Lab Considered

The Lean Six Sigma Process Improvement team has drafted a proposal to streamline work productivity from the laboratory personnel by just moving the entire space to the smoke deck.

In lieu of no one ever actually being in the lab spaces when they are needed, Role 3 leadership is seriously considering the initiative.

Spearheaded by the entire Nurse Corps of the hospital, the space left behind where the lab used to be would be the newly constructed safe space where they may gather and cry about being bullied by doctors or disrespected by ancillary services.

The DCSS Director is fighting for this change because he misses cage-fighting back in Hawaii. "If you're not fighting for your people, it's time to leave or die," he allegedly said.

Page 2 VOL: I ISSUE: II

WHISKEY SAILOR NEARS RECORD, CAN'T REMEMBER OWN NAME

In an extreme act of bravery, there is one Petty Officer who has risen above the rest, and is now paying the price for his sacrifice.

No one of consequence can recall the last time HM3 Jimmy Writer left the hospital, and he is beginning to forget his own name as a direct result of the dedication shown in the service of his country.

If it weren't for Petty Officer Writer's boyish charm and looks, his facial hair would look something out of a bad comedy film.

Possibly if Writer was less

Because copyright.

Most recent picture of HM3 Writer

concerned with the patients under his care and more with his own well-being, he would actually look normal.

What is most interesting about the position HM3 has placed himself in is the Iron-man record he is currently chasing of most days consecutively spent at KAF Role 3 MMU.

Previously held by then-Chief Lorenzo Branch of Beatty, MO, it is a record that most feel was untouchable. It is also a record that no one wants.

"It's like baseball's hit-by-pitch record or the NFL interception record," cites one lesser mortal, "no one wants that kind of notoriety, but someone also has to have it."

Writer is clearly putting himself in a position to be driven as a Clydesdale when he's more of a "Lil Sebastian" type. May we tip our caps for the Writers of Whiskey because it's Sailors like him which keep the Navy in safe hands for the future years.

What he cannot do is very different from what he won't do.

SUPPO REFUSES TO PLACE CAREER ON LINE

"Back when I got in, we used Sears Catalogs, and even that was charity."

Don't expect the bare necessities like two-ply toilet paper while LCDR Warner is calling the shots. The Supply Officer for Whiskey Rotation is not taking any chances to ruin his retirement package from the Navy. The crusty veteran isn't sympathetic to the candy-asses of NATO's newest medical unit either. He may have said that, "back when I got in, we used Sears catalogs, and even that was charity."

No doubt the Butt Floss Boss came in when ships were still primarily powered by the wind, but contracts are contracts and they can't be breached for nobody. His lack of empathy is causing a ruckus within the ranks.

One Filipino Chief said that he's got cousins who can do SUPPO's job and still have time to gain an organized "crime" reputation.

At the end of the day, we can all enjoy the multi-wipes, swamp ass and chocolate covered fingers for a few months longer because of one man's decision to only think about himself and his flakey cigars.

ROLE 3 REP FOR KAF COMPETITIVE EATING TOURNAMENT ANNOUNCED

At a recent Role 3 Leadership briefing, the rational decision to select LCDR Claudine Bansil as the Role 3 representative for the 4th of July Competitive Eating Contest was announced.

It has been reported that Mrs. Bansil is heavily training by raiding all the good snacks which is provided in the galley fridge and other night staff's secret coffers.

There may be fierce competition, but as long as

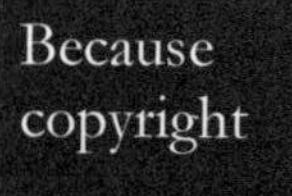

Kobeyashi remains one of the world's greatest there is hope for the ICU nurse to flourish in this challenge.

The winner will earn a firm handshake from the KAF Commanding General and LOA from the Role 3 CO. Please inquire with PS2 Krombach for more information.

Ran out of ideas, filler pic here

LaPenna dreams of stacking bodies, pokes IV fluid bags instead

Combat Pharmacy Technician Michael LaPenna wanted to join the Marines because he, "wanted to know what it was like to kill somebody."

Fate is a cruel mistress to reality though, and he has ended up being trained to save the lives he once wanted to mercilessly end as a Hospital Corpsman.

The killers edge has never left the salty Sailor since he was recently seen taking his frustrations out on 125 boxes, or 1,345 bags of expired IV fluids from a local connex box.

From once wanting to stack bodies to now poking holes can be a humbling transition for any man or woman. There was a palpable feeling of growing frustration when the Thirsty Camel came to visit the Bag Slayer.

Upon further investigation, it became obvious that there was more than a killer's instinct at play. Slicing and dicing over a thousand bags as the most senior E6 certainly is humbling, but when you are doing it with your dumb ass Second Class, it tests the limits of a man.

Whatever the mission, wherever the call is made, the role of the combat pharmacy will never diminish, waiver or fade. It rises to the highest levels of service our country calls for and will deal with the most difficult of nurses. HM1 LaPenna is a shining example of discipline to rate, and what one may come if more selflessness was brought to the work place.

"I wanted to join the Marines so I could find out what it was like to kill somebody."

LCDR Stewart knows what he wants to be for Halloween

An Emergency Department nurse has already decided what he wants to be for Halloween, whether he is still stuck in KAF or not.

Lieutenant Commander John Stewart, despite having one of the most boring, yet most well-known names ever, wants to take his Night of Horrors into a different direction by trying to pull off the "Anderson Cooper" look.

Stewart believes that as long as he can keep his mouth shut and refrain from attempting to sound intelligent, the costume could be a massive hit.

Halloween is scheduled for 31 October 2020 this year, a radical shift from years past.

Sir looks like Anderson Cooper, change my mind

"LCDR Stewart"

Neurosurgeon the loneliest sailor

CDR Cooke has it very rough. On one hand he is too young to fit into Whiskey's "Good 'ol Boys" Club of the other ancient surgeons, but too old to considered cool for the JO's. He is too smart to want the XO's job, and too green to assume command.

We should all feel bad for the only reason why we consider ourselves a "Role 3" medical facility. We should feel this way because when he goes home he doesn't have a roommate to hang out, to talk about his day. He has all that empty space in that room of his, by himself, but no one to perform activities with.

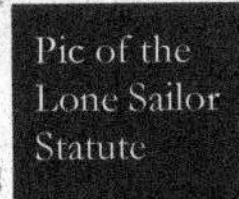

Anything less than lamenting CDR Cooke's plot in life would be uncivilized. So what if he looks like Ivan Drago's cousin when he's in the middle of a hunger strike?

Yes, indeed, you would be lonely too if you had to work with HM2 Drumheller everyday. No amount of spiked hair will get him to fit in, and if there's one thing to learn as a cautionary tale it's that the devil wears Prada, or so it's been told.

Tekashi 6ix9ine to Rewrite Navy Song

As part of a court-mandated 300 hours of community service, " musical artist" Daniel Hernandez, must rewrite the Navy theme song of "Anchors Away." Mr. Hernandez is known to the world as "Tekashi 6ix9ine."

The flamboyant and highly disturbed individual has recently been accused of racketeering, firearms and drug trafficking, but is just what Department of Navy

A national treasure pictured here.

Tekashi 6ix9ine

brass is looking for.

"We need to bring a newer new Navy," says one top gun official, "6ix9ine brings a fresh face to our recruiting platform. He's bold and takes chances. We want to see more of that from our enlisted force. Plus, he came at a discount, and you know how the bean counters are with saving money in these times."

The anchors aren't so sure. Rumor has it the newcomer is recognized as a serious threat among the Goat Locker to its time honored traditions.

One Sandy Goat said, "If someone is going to look stupid and break the rules, it's going to be us." The source later said, "I'll like the new song only if it mentions Hennessy or Patron. Beer is good too, but a good one like Miller High Life. You know, the champagne of beers."

Whiskey Helps

RADIOLOGIST SEES SHADOW, GOES BACK TO HIDING FOR 6 MORE WEEKS

Whiskey Rotation radiologist Dr. Paul Cripe has seen his shadow this past Tuesday, and has decided it would be becoming of his role in the hospital to go back into hiding for six more weeks.

LCDR Cripe is following a rich line of Role 3 MMU radiology traditionalists which states that whenever they see the light of the Sun, a rapid-fire decision must be made as to be exposed to the world or not. By way of this tradition, every radiologist since Charlie rotation has run into hiding never to be seen.

There is often much speculation as to what a radiologist does with their time. One combat laboratory technician could only guess. "Well, they are never on the smoke deck because that's where we are," they were heard to say. One radiology technician sensed that his department head was being attacked, but had to press pause on their video game to give an accurate quote.

"We are very busy over here saving lives."

No doubt in anyone's mind. Good luck, sir!

RASTALL AND FREDDIE TRYOUT FOR WWE

Petty Officer Rastall and Logistic Technician "Freddie" have submitted videotape to the WWE in the hopes to tryout for the next Table, Ladders, and Chairs Pay-Per-View match this winter. Rumor has it they will be reprising the "Dudley Boyz" gimmick and have been practicing afterhours in the supply warehouse. Using Eugene as a placeholder, they have been climbing to the top of the shelves and fine-tuning their flying elbows and Won-Ton Swan dives. Rastall especially is jacked to finally find a friendly rival. Sean allows it, but we can't go near his desk. Sports Entertainment is not fake, it's predetermined.

Two guys here who liked to go get the tables. Because copyright.

WOOLEN SHOTGUNS CASE OF WHOOP ASS, CALLS LORD RAIDEN A "BITCH"

In dramatic fashion, HM1 David Woolen has entered into the centennial Mortal Kombat tournament by calling out 10x defending champion, God of Thunder, Lord Raiden.

The insanity supposedly started after a rare mistake in Amazon Prime's logistics algorithm and shipped an entire pallet of Whoop Ass energy drinks to the admin paper pusher.

Not believing the luck which fell unto the unsuspecting Petty Officer, Woolen then decided to go on an all-night bender with Captain Insano's heavily endorsed beverage of the gods. It was reported that there was a lot of emphasis on meeting an arbitrary deadline set by someone with an anchor and no common sense.

By the break of dawn, HM1 had consumed enough Whoop Ass to stimulate a corpse from across the River Styx. In a

Picture of Lord Raiden here. No money or need to purchase license to use photo. Would rather make joke

Lord Raiden, 10x Mortal Komat Champion

moment of an absolute loss of sanity, the gauntlet was thrown and called Lord Raiden a "bitch," He was consequently challenged in the next Mortal Kombat tournament which ironically takes place later this year.

Growing up in the shadow of Jesse Pinkman, Woolen is familiar with getting his ass kicked, but feels this time he will have the high ground.

"Whoop Ass leaves any opponent shown no mercy," mumbled the focused, soon to be utterly destroyed First Class.

Lord Raiden could not be reached at his local tabernacle. His harem of dimes took the message.

Mortal Kombat is a competition between the two realms which takes place once every 100 years. Its story is legendary, spinning off into multiple video games and one decent live action film. A follow-up film, Mortal Kombat: Annihilation was about as piss poor as a movie can be and is often disregarded as canon.

You may be ugly as Goro, but FINISH HIM!!, HM1 and may the odds ever be in your favor.

9 June 2020
Day 113

Another 24-hour duty, and another close to the day. I'm very tired, but still have a couple things to do like temperature checks, bag expired meds, and write one more piece for *The Whiskey Ration.* Hopefully it will all be fast.

My day was nothing special except that I finished Issue #2 of *The Thirsty Camel.* So far my worst fear hasn't happened, and that was tanking it on my second outing. With the element of surprise lost, could I pull it off again? It seems like I have, so far. *The Thirsty Camel* is very time consuming for my thoughts and that's good and bad.

I've been logging a lot of time with HM1 LaPenna too, and I think that is good. His hustle and general pharmacy technician knowledge are very beneficial to me. We are still getting closer to understanding one another in terms of leadership perspective and theory, but I haven't had one bad conversation with him yet, and that is motivating.

I don't think I'll be reading my book tonight, but I could always surprise myself. I could get over myself at any time and get sweaty again. No one cares about a little knee pain or general soreness. No one cares, it's okay to be hungry, and if I'm so smart, why aren't I winning?

Postscript: That last paragraph had some "isms" I picked up on the deployment. Strangely enough, they were all from one person. I would like to show that I was always thinking about it and listening to what was said. LaPenna is a guy who I truly liked, and it is unfortunate that it did not always seem that way. We had a common bond by both being previously stationed on an aircraft carrier. He was on the USS Abraham Lincoln (CVN-72) and I was on the USS Theodore Roosevelt (CVN-71). We could always resort to the "good old days," and it helped take our minds off the bad times.

12 June 2020
Day 114, 115 & 116

This entry is a bit of a big deal to me because by the final day I will have written in every page of this journal. That's right, I've completed this journal and it's actually a real sense of accomplishment. Now we'll just have to transcribe this little by little. If I could access Google Docs on these government computers that would be awesome. Until then, I'll just bring my Chromebook in and flip it open when it gets slow.

Unlike last night when we had four patients arrive. To my happy surprise, we've only had one American patient so far, to my knowledge, and it was for some minor reason. I guess yesterday there was an active shooter somewhere off base. The shooter and three victims came in. That's the thing with these patients though, especially the host nation (Afghan) military.

An episode of *Reading Rainbow* doesn't have this much imagination to its stories. I guess we currently have an Afghan general that survived an assassination attempt, and there is a credible threat that there are those who want to infiltrate the base, gain access to the hospital, and finish the job. The idea sounds crazy, and I don't know what to think. I know that he is the reason why I spend so much time in the fume hood.

Today I was there for two and a half hours making IVs for everyone. That sucked, but once it was over I had most of my day.

We, LCDR Fitzgerald and I, had a good collaboration in getting the newsletter complete. Our regular layout editor, HM3 Writer, was selected for Motivator of the Month, and we gave him the issue off. He has been working very hard on many projects, so I think he could have needed the break. My Hospital Corpsman article made the cut. It's a reprise of an article jointly written with my good friend Caleb Ellis. It was first published in Iwakuni, and I have always wanted to reuse it. I'm satisfied that the opportunity presented itself.

Tonight, I wrote three letters, and it was the stress-reliever I needed. My penmanship was on point, the words just flowed, it felt great. My dad got a letter and so did Aaron Eastman, and Alex Schmidt's family too. All three were one page each, but with free postage I can get away with that.

Lately I have been spending more time at work exercising the Golden Rule. If I see work that needs to be done, I help. For one, HM1 Wilson is about as comfortable in the fume hood as I should be proficient in it. The only tech who truly carries his share of their load, and then some, for technician duties is HM1 LaPenna. I can only try to keep up. His hustle is truly inspiring. HM1 Wilson did however teach me a little trick with formatting memos. It had to deal with adjusting the tab spacing. Needless to say, I was pretty jazzed and look forward to the next memo I need to write.

Really, I wanted to know how I could knock the rust off my correspondence skills. In the meantime, not only did I do that, but I also crafted a piece of correspondence to the Commanding Officer. I was not happy with our mass communication crisis management system. My recommendation was to use what USNH Yokosuka and its branch clinics use, Blackberry AtHoc. Who knows how it'll turn out, probably in failure, but as HM1 Levi Arcaira taught me, things can still be learned in failure. I find that encouraging.

Haven't listened to my book in a few days, but that's because I haven't exercised. Was going to jog this morning, but yeah. I'm still listening to Stephen King's *On Writing* and I just passed the 100th page of *Dr. Sleep.* Typical King, fast read, but can get really bizarre in a hurry.

Tomorrow is laundry day at self-serve and a new journal.

Postscript: A couple of things to unpack. I understood I was the weakest link in the pharmacy and therefore the biggest liability. No one explicitly said it, but for the entire time I was there I felt inferior to who I stood beside. From my four previous duty stations to Afghanistan, I had never had to do inpatient care, and for the most part it was the entire reason I was needed. Luckily, I had help, and regrettably I did not always show my appreciation. It should also be noted that when I spoke of patients, there was a high chance I was regurgitating the latest, racist rumor about that patient. I never knew their real names. Every patient, at least Afghan, were given an alias for not only their protection, but ours too.

14 Jun 2020
Day 117 & 118

Oh, what times we live in. Technically it is 0440 on the 15th of June. I went to bed early so that I could wake up early to do things out of the sun.

First up on today's menu is my laundry. They have taken all but one bench away so I'm using my lap as a table. It's alright because I have my new journal I'm writing in. It's almost a shame the readers on the internet or computer print format will never get to truly know or see the sense and magnitude of my accomplishment.

Today is going to be the day I start working out again, but this journal records what has happened versus the future prophecies. Yesterday was a bit of a whirlwind. I went to sleep early two nights ago too, but I couldn't stay sleeping. That's why last night I took 75mg of Benadryl, and it worked. Anyway, I was "awake" from about 2230 to 0400 and was so mad at myself. I just stayed in bed. The whole time I kept thinking to myself that if I'm going to be awake, I should at least get something out of it. Instead, I continued to flip through Instagram. It almost felt cowardly.

I slept from 0400 until called by HM1 Wilson at 1030 telling me that I needed to cover for HM1 LaPenna. It wasn't clear to me at the moment, but when LaPenna covered for me on my command duty day, I told him I would return the favor. Today was that day, and I blew it by forgetting. I did hustle to the hospital though in personal record time and sat on the computer.

A good chunk of *The Thirsty Camel* was complete. I'm beginning to imagine a world where the *Camel* doesn't exist. I think there will be one or two people who will write somewhere to someone that they have a problem with it and that'll be a wrap. Such times we live in.

COVID-19 is now firmly present in Kandahar, Afghanistan. There is little hope the gym will ever reopen in our time here. That makes me incredibly sad. All the shops around the boardwalk are now permanently closed, but a part of that might be planned. They might have been looking for a good time to close as part of the pull-out plan, and they found it.

Drumheller has gotten me turned onto a new Netflix show called *F is for Family* (2015). It's rather vulgar, but very funny. It was created by Bill Burr, and I would compare it to a cross of *Life with Louie* (1994), *The Simpsons* (1989), and a Seth McFarlane production.

Overall, life is consistent here.

Postscript: Stress was high on my deployment. Maybe the imminent threat of an offensive by the bad guys was not as present as earlier rotations, but I always wanted to do the right thing. We depended on one another so much, and when I let a teammate down because I "forgot," that was an excuse that made me feel even worse. I think everyone had their weird way of getting away from it all, and for me it was doing my own laundry. We had laundry service at the hospital where we could drop off our bags and the next day they would be ready for pickup, but when I was at the self-service no one talked to me, and I wasn't rushed. Honestly, it was one of my favorite places to go when I wanted to be alone.

15 Jun 2020
Day 119

Today is one of my 24-hour shifts. I felt productive and can go to bed feeling fulfilled. If I could do one more thing, it would be to transcribe some journal entries, but that might be asking for too much.

I am a page deep in my LGBT speech with about a page to go. I did pushups today as promised with Freddie and the boys. Only did 50 and I felt almost every one of them.

My cigarette total has risen to six since leaving Japan. I don't feel that good about it. The command climate survey came out today, just in time for Issue #3 of *The Thirsty Camel.* We are calling it the "Pre-DEOCS" issue. I am predicting that *The Thirsty Camel* will be brought to an abrupt halt after the results come out.

Called home and the boys were so good, lying-in bed like a couple of angels. Mail Call today. Someone shipped a five-pound bag of coffee to me, but I'm not sure who. Maybe Shuhei Hamaguchi, but I told a few people to mail coffee, so who knows. No letters, yet. I'll keep knocking them out as they still relax me writing them.

It was a good day.

Postscript: In the pharmacy, we had a coffee maker and electric water kettle. We never used the water kettle, but we abused the hell out of the coffee pot. Sure, we had some coffee, but when your coworker back in Sasebo is straight Cuban, you tend to be spoiled a little bit. I missed that, and when that coffee came in, I was so appreciative I immediately wrote a thank you card to the barista. Moreover, since then I have only bought Enderley Coffee from North Carolina. The coffee wars between the departments on who had the best brew became a bit of a big deal. Because the pharmacy was a locked space, it was not able to enter the unofficial competition.

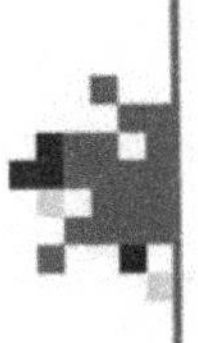

THE THIRSTY CAMEL

DEFINITELY NOT A NATO ROLE 3 MMU PUBLICATION

Volume 1, Issue 3

"The pre-DEOCS Survey Edition"

FUN DAY SCHEDULED FOR ED

Emergency Department Leadership wants to award all the hard work and dedication to the mission for all of its staff. They are said to be scheduling an outing "fun day," and cutting out early for the day.

"We are the first line of defense to saving a life here at KAF," spouted one larger than life ED physician, "Our focus is 100% spent on the welfare of the department we are billeted for."

The Fun Day should not be without some controversy however marginal. The Chiefs Mess is all for this morale event. Says one USN bearer, "ED has all those Corpsmen. They need to exercise those lungs and give their eyes a rest after watching all those educational movies in the dark."

Anti-funny pic of a man coined "the comedian."

"For a guy who calls yourself a comedian, Camel, I can never tell when you are being funny."

Sources say that the memo written to the Skipper excludes the ICU staff, citing, " they don't have any Corpsmen anyway and 'Negative Nancys 'bum' them out."

Clinical Support Services are issuing a self-imposed ban because they actually have work to do.

Except HM2 Terrell, who is not only invited, but has somehow word-smithed himself as a deputy organizer.

The memo went on to demand manning coverage in their absence from the most qualified department, the ICU.

INSIDE THIS ISSUE:

Doctor does time	2
Stolen Valor	2
Band Lifecycle	2
Bronze Star Media	3
Muffin Man Met	3
Word Wars	3
PS2 Awarded	4
Room Failure	4

SPECIAL POINTS OF INTEREST:

- The Thirsty Camel is released whenever the publisher damn well feels like it good and proper.
-

THE CAMEL GOES TO CHURCH

The Thirsty Camel went to Church the other day. Believe him, he knows all about DEOCS Surveys. When he should probably be more concerned with getting railroaded and ultimately cancelled, that isn't what it prayed for.

May the axes that need to be grinded be done so justly, and with objectivity. He hopes any rage be tempered, first world problems managed, and what truly matters become recognized. Stupid questions do exist, but unfortunately so do false realties.

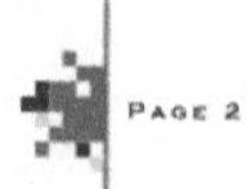

Photo of 0.0% Amstel Beer we cherished

INTENSIVIST DETAINED BY KAF PROVOST MARSHAL OFFICE

Captain Kahler did not get much sleep this past Tuesday night after picking up LCDR Salazar from the KAF base security Provost Marshal's Office.

Alleged documentation cites the ICU physician as being detained by PMO after refusing to show identification for walking out of the Monti DFAC with two Amstel "near beers."

Said one PMO official, "It is base policy to be at least 18 years old to obtain even 'non-alcoholic' beer." The source went on to say, "my comrades had to release the doctor because she did a solid helping my cousin Igor."

Mrs. Salazar spent three hours in the interrogation room, but was finally released after correctly answering who Finkel is.

"Only someone who is of age would be able to answer that riddle."

Regardless, Dr. Salazar now has to cover for CAPT Kahler's next three duties.

"ONLY ONE VOICE CAN PULL OFF THE "GOOD MORNING VIETNAM" HAPPINESS, AND WE DON'T EXPECT ROBIN WILLIAMS TO REPRISE HIS ROLE ANY TIME SOON,"

ANNOYING VOICE IN SKY CHARGED WITH STOLEN VALOR

That annoying voice Role 3 gets to hear every morning has been found and charged with stolen valor.

"Only one voice can pull off the "Good Morning Vietnam" happiness, and we don't expect Robin Williams to reprise his role any time soon," said one Romanian serviceman.

It is true, since the world lost its favorite military DJ, there has been many copycats, and all have failed to live up to the ridiculous standard set by Williams.

KAF's turn at disappointment has taken on its own brand of disservice to a man's memory though, and the base brass is taking action on rectifying an already sad situation.

All I want for Christmas is to not get sued. Insert Mariah Carey holiday album cover here.

LIFECYCLE OF YOUR FAVORITE BAND

Have you ever wondered what happened to your favorite band or musician? Fear not because the Thirsty Camel staff has developed the musician lifecycle for your viewing pleasure.

First is commercial fame. They are on the radio more than our ears can handle and after a few tours and albums, they decide to "give back" to the troops. This is the first signs of a slow death.

After the USO Tour, they will release a couple more albums no one will listen to, and in a final grasp for being a shell of themselves, the inevitable Christmas album will be released. Think about it.

SEARCH FOR BRONZE STAR MEDIA COVERAGE CONTINUES

Victor rotation's unprecedented end of tour awards has yet to gain the attention of not one Public Affairs Office or third party media source.

A single Bronze Star within a unit is a notable achievement, but Victor Rotation produced no less than 12 recipients and no one is talking about it.

The rumor is that no one, from the Armed Forces Network , Navy Times to the Inspector General would believe the report should it ever see the light of day on their desks.

"If Whiskey Rotation can be known for one thing, it is that they uphold the "Bro Code" and don't narc out their 'bros,' even if they are the most passive aggressive unit since that "Mean Girls" movie," allegedly said one thinly-haired senior officer.

These are unbelievable times only meant for fictitious satire newsletters, yet here we are. Stay strong, Whiskey, and keep your stick on the ice.

A picture of a thing you'll get for preparation of the worst pandemic since Spanish Flu and not actually in the trenches with it.

PHARMACY CLAIMS TO HAVE MET THE MUFFIN MAN

We all know the children's movie "Shrek" and the scene, where the gingerbread man is being tortured. He's asked by an over-compensating Lord Farquad the location of the fat ogre.

In a final attempt to shed the vertically challenged tormentor, Farquad is asked if he knows who the Muffin Man is. You know, the one on Drury Lane.

Great news Whiskey drinkers! The staff of your very own pharmacy has claimed, on good authority, to have not only seen, but met the homemade-delicious man.

In unrelated news, the Controlled Substance Inventory Board is working full tilt backtracking on the location of all the benzos.

"YOU KNOW, THE ONE ON DRURY LANE."

WAR OVER PROPER SPELLING OF ABBREVIATED MASS CASUALTY

Some debate has been lingering within the ranks as to what to short-hand a Mass Casualty. Around some water coolers, it is MASCAS and around other campfires it is pronounced MASCAL.

You do not need to be Elon Musk to know that it is MASCAS. Much like we say MEDEVAC for MEDical EVACuation.

Of course there is only good order and discipline here at Whiskey, and we will continue to pretend along if it should otherwise be pronounced differently.

It should be noted that the leaders of the MASCAL movement are indeed from California...and Montana.

"I JUST CAN'T GET BEHIND IT. IT LITERALLY SOUNDS LIKE SOMEONE CHEWING WITH THEIR PIE-HOLE OPEN...IS THIS THE PSYCHOLOGICAL WARFARE THEY'RE ALWAYS TALKING ABOUT IN THE MILITARY?"

-HM1 LAPENNA

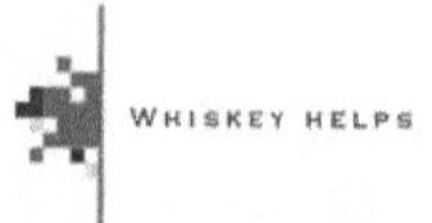

WILCOX AND KENTUCKIAN IN 2ND PLACE

Long-time Officers of the United States Navy Reserve LT Ben Wilcox and someone from Kentucky are now in the first runner up spot for Roommates of the Rotation after failing a recent room inspection.

Documents obtained by the Thirsty Camel state that the hits for failing ranged everything from CPAP hoses adrift to improperly stowed bottles of Gerirol and Manup.

This room inspection may come as a surprise because it only happens to the peons stuck with a roommate, nothing that any E3's would know something about.

"I guess commissioned officers don't get theirs, but kids in "Chief billets" do," observed one Whiskey staffer, "at least the pay guy is happy, and if he's happy, chances are I might be too."

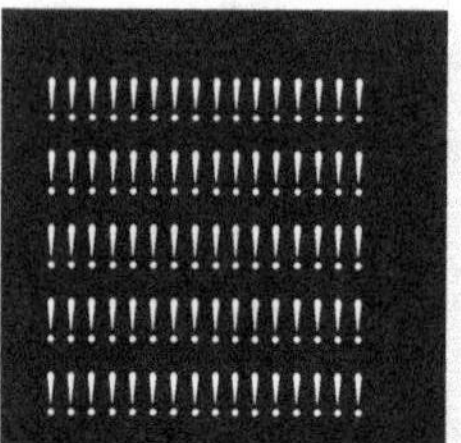

Should Krombach ever ride into war, his shield shall bear this marking.

HARDCORE PHYSICIAN SLATED TO JOIN WHISKEY

In order to help release the growing tension, Whiskey's Skipper has reached out and hired a hardcore physician. Coming later this month, Dr. Jonathan Sins of Bel Air Mercy Hospital is expected to report. Upon hearing the news, some staff are going to be able to manage with another doctor in the house. Dr. Sins comes very qualified and is ready to please the team he's assigned with. He comes with a solid package of credentials and stiff bedside manner, but will certainly rise to the occasion when summoned by the head nurse.

> Dr. Sins has a license on his image even though he gave me a Cameo shout-out. #facts.

Wilson uses Pretend Names to Produce make-believe Titles

The Leading Petty Officer of the Clinical Support Services Directorate has gone rogue and given himself a new title: God's Gift to the Navy.

In a recent email that was sent to directorate staff, he ordered that all subordinates and peers address him as such.

This news comes in the wake of a slew of other Sailors coming up with own titles to juke their stats, alter reality, and farm the best eval possible. Subordinate pharmacy tech, HM2 Rastall, also wishes to be addressed as: King Neptune's General Counsel, a nod probably referring to his penchant to sea-lawyering.

LCDR Deguzman was not available to comment because he was busy training for the next cage fight held at KAF later this summer.

KROMBACH IS MOST EFFICIENT

Whiskey Rotation's Pay Boss has been recently recognized as the most efficient Sailor in the unit.

PS2 Robert Krombach has garnered the most attention, accolades and perks for literally moving the least of anyone in the unit. His movement to production ratio is off the charts and it deserves the type of recognition fitting for someone in their position.

Not even the Chiefs move as little as PS2 does, they are at least pounding the deckplates and shipmating.

The extent of his work productivity may appear to be the click of a mouse and some emails sent, but it's the results of what he gets from doing all that labor.

Remarkably, he's been able to shed weight despite his desk job, maybe because he only eats half his wings at a time.

You know you're on his good side when you get at least three exclamation points in a single standard email. Anything less is the mark of a shot across the bow.

Petty Officer is not deaf, dumb or inconsiderate with his grammar, he's just from New York, and we should extend his leash a little farther.

Krombach Day will entail us not shaving like him, so sign the petition today.

16 Jun 2020
Day 120

Now I'm sore, again. If I hate this feeling, why would I allow myself to go back to it? This morning I exercised legitimately at the Swole 3 gym in the back of the hospital. I'll save what I did in my workout for a different journal, but I did get in 100 pushups, in total. My back hurts more than my chest for some reason.

Anyway, it caused me to start my morning off on the right foot, and I was pretty productive from 0630 to 0830 when HM1 Wilson got into work. I made that new cup of coffee that was delivered yesterday, and it was delicious. To confirm, it was Hamaguchi, and he recommended I write a letter to the owners of the coffee store. That is exactly what I did with my first cup still in hand.

I called Saori, too. I've been neglecting her needs lately and had time to talk to her about Explore Translation matters. It was a very nice call. When I called tonight, I was reasonably expecting the boys, but Okasan put them to bed already and I guess I couldn't hide the disappointment in my face very well. It made Saori laugh.

We had one patient arrive today. Apparently, either one or many sandbags fell on his head. He was talking when I last saw him. An ICU nurse gave a day's worth of propranolol to the patient at one time. His 10mg QID, four times a day, was taken together. He'll live, and hopefully not a sign of karma.

Postscript: As a pharmacy technician, I can admit that medical mistakes happen more often than we would like to admit. Normally they are of the same severity as what happened above, but sometimes the wrong leg is sawed off. Medicine is practiced for a reason, and it is a continuous evolution of process improvement. If a baseball player hits a ball 40% of the time throughout their career, they are headed straight to the hall of fame. If a medical professional is less than 100% correct, they are sued, and that is the world we live in. Not saying it's right or wrong, but it hopefully offers some perspective.

18 Jun 2020
Days 121 & 122

Holy cow what a past couple of days this has been. It's actually 0030 on the 19th, and I'm still looking at an hour or two of consistent work ahead of me.

Before that though, there are some things I should share. First of all, happy belated birthday Hospital Corps. You're 122 years young. After 12 short years of service to the United States Navy, I finally held a meaningful position as the Master of Ceremonies. I felt it could have gone better, but as HM1 Wilson assured me, I'm always going to be my worst critic.

Although I was sore, I went to the track that night. After 120 pushups and 2 miles jogging, and one mile walking I'm beginning to realize I don't get that "runner's high." In fact, I felt awful afterward, but I put in a good effort. I'm just excited for this effort to pay off.

My roommate, HM2 Drumheller, did not attend the HM Birthday presentation, and I was more hurt than anything. I would have gone to whatever thing he was the Master of Ceremonies for even if I felt differently about it.

I called the boys tonight and felt like I was actually talking to Josiah. I asked him to show me a book he liked, and he went upstairs to show me *The Giving Tree*. We sang songs, he identified colors and knew how many fingers I was holding up. Man, it meant so much to me, and I can't wait to be home again.

Especially after the foot-in-mouth situation I had today. The details can be spared here because it is not something I like thinking about. I'm very embarrassed at myself. What I did was lose sight of self-control and misread situational awareness. It was something that I'll be thinking about for a long time. One day I hope to forgive myself.

Then there is the patient that refuses to live, but modern medicine is refusing to let die. Our general from Afghanistan who was shot in the face. The odds of his survival will not be anything less than a miracle. He began crashing and seizing about an hour after LCDR Deguzman left, and he was essentially recalled back.

He and I worked until about 2300 straight. I asked him if he would still be coming in had the far superior tech, HM1 LaPenna, been working. He said that he would; a man was dying. I guess that made me feel a little better. This self-image problem I have is getting a little ridiculous. I wonder how much of it is tied to my weight. My guess is a lot. Ugh! Such a slow process!

I'm almost done with my Stephen King memoir *On Writing*. It's enjoyable, but I'm ready to move on to the next Audible title.

So much left to do. Gotta get to work.

Postscript: There it is, and I just glossed right over it, sandwiching it between every other inconsequential bit of news. That conversation I was embarrassed about still haunts me to this day and glooms over my reflection of Whiskey Rotation*. For me, everything changed after that moment. I still will not share what was said, or who was involved, but it was the lowest point I had ever been in a professional setting. I don't like being reminded of it, I don't like thinking about it, and I don't like sharing it, but there it was. I've said a lot of stupid things to the wrong person many times over, but not like that suspended moment in time. What was done is done, and in case everyone else forgot about it, no fear because I will carry that boat for a long time.*

20 Jun 2020
Days 123 & 124

I wish there was more to report over the past two days, but there just isn't. I am writing before going to the track where I have beat myself, or lack thereof, for the past two days. Almost felt it last night, but decided to snuggle in with my book instead.

That should mean I was actually reading my book, but what it truly meant was I had the intention of reading, but sat on my phone until late into the night instead. It's behavior like that which pisses me off, and how I blow so many opportunities of productivity.

While I'm at it, I officially hate my desk. It's too short to get underneath, my thighs that is, and it's too dark here in the corner of the room. It may sound like I'm in a bad mood, but I don't feel like I'm in one.

Because of scheduling, I decided to do my Father's Day thing a day early. I recorded myself reading a book and sent it to the boys. It was "sponsored" by the MWR. If you count them supplying the book, then yeah, they were hugely instrumental in making this happen. My only true regret was the video couldn't be more than five minutes long or the file is too large to send.

That was almost the most exciting part of my day because it was my day off. I slept until 1030, again. I went to bed at 0100, but I keep surprising myself. Woke up, watched the new Netflix show *Space Force* (2020) with Steve Carrell and went back to sleep for a couple hours. My roommate, HM2 Justin Drumheller, came home at about 1330. We watched a couple episodes of *F is for Family* (2015), and then I left the room.

Sadly, I bought my first pack of cigarettes. HM1 LaPenna made fun of me because they were Pall Mall Reds. I don't blame him, and as of today I need to turn off the nicotine counter.

Also got my haircut today. Asked for the Greg Fall special, bald as it can be without a razor blade.

Maybe I need to write a letter or two; that might help. Christina Solomon called today. We rescheduled for tomorrow evening though. It was nice seeing a familiar face again though.

This last portion is more of a postscript. I walked away from my desk, plugged my headphones into the charger and sat on my phone. If I wasn't much of a jabroni, I wouldn't have minded. There I was, on my phone into the late hours and didn't return to finish this until later into the night.

It was the first time I don't recall having anything to say. Oh well, tomorrow is another day, and may it never happen again. I'm better than this.

Postscript: I didn't have my first beer until the night I graduated high school. It was in the garage of my Uncle Gordie. I didn't smoke a cigarette until my swimming career was finished. I chewed tobacco almost consistently for 10 years. I thought it was a good time to quit dipping when my 3-year-old son would hand me my spit bottle when I never even asked for it. Nicorette chewing gum is much more socially acceptable, and working in the pharmacy, I had a direct link to supply. Not knowing what the situation was going to be like in Afghanistan, I quit on the way over. If a person is the average of the five people you spend the most time with, I was doomed to start smoking again.

21 Jun 2020
Day 125

Happy Father's Day. Wouldn't you know that today is my 24-hour shift. I think a lot happened today, but it was all routine in many ways too.

Of course, I didn't work out like I promised myself I would. I did however get to work not rushed and showered. When I got to the office, I wrapped up Issue #4 of *The Thirsty Camel.* What I've been noticing is that *The Camel* has been saturating the market. Although the content remains good, it's not getting the desired pop I crave. In other words, it's no longer a scarce item and I need to slow it down.

We placed boxes of unusable fluids beneath a Ford 750 truck and "drained" them that way. It felt like *A River Runs Through It* for some reason to me, and I wrote the following in a group chat:

For a suspended moment in time, we were there, separated from differences, struggles and confusion. It was here we were young again and into the night we knew it was going to be okay.

Possibly the best compliment I received in a long time came from HM2 Jed Rodriguez who asked if I plagiarized that from a book. Of course, I didn't, and I think that was his way of acknowledging that.

Dad was gone fishing when I called. Jonica and Grandma Mongin were over though. Calling Dr. Christina "Dearest" was enriching.

Postscript: That was a fond memory. We all got wet with salty normal saline as it exploded beneath the weight of that truck. We had fun; there were lots of laughs. It wasn't the first time A River Runs Through It *crossed my mind over this deployment. As the Afghan sun was setting, and the longing of home beared down on our souls, we did something together, and it made all the difference.*

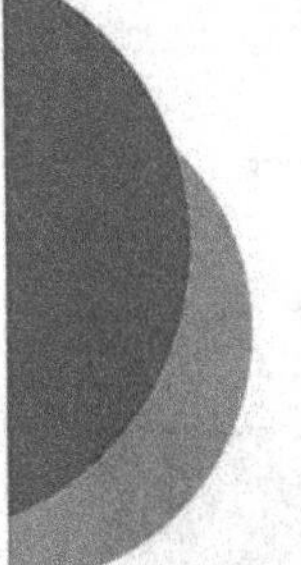

The Thirsty Camel

Volume I, Issue 4 Published: Precisely When it was Meant To

Definitely Not a Role 3 MMU Publication

Special points of interest:

- Keep your words soft and sweet in case you have to eat them.
- If you hear anyone say there is no such thing as a perfect Sailor, they clearly have met HM1 Wilson.
- When you read the Thirsty Camel you are misinformed. When you don't, you're uninformed.
- HM2 Slagle's mustache has a name and it's David Pretzel.
- Brophy, this isn't 'Nam, this is KAF, there are rules.

Inside this issue:

SEL Gets Crazy	2
Camel Editorial	2
Workshop for Nurses	2
DMS Getting Swole	3
Message to PAD	3
Nicest of Them All	3
2nd Class Dual	4
Fatherland Pride	4

SEA CONFUSED OVER SECOND PLACE, ASSERTS PRIVILEGE

Role 3 enlisted are standing by for heavy rolls as the Senior Enlisted Advisor is working through some serious shit.

At the last First Class Petty Officer Meeting, the rotation's Leprechaun was voted on, and the vertically challenged most senior enlisted was not mentioned in the final round of nominations.

Rotation Leprechaun is a prestigious collateral position given to a Role 3 MMU Sailor who is decidedly the most deserving according to the top of the bottom of enlisted ranks. Although the specific guidance remains unwritten and mysterious on the selection process, anyone is typically fair game.

HM2 Anthony Roberts has been chosen as the unit's lucky Leprechaun, and his selection has been met with high praise across the deckplates.

"Roberts is as tall as a sugary cereal mascot, has a laugh about as appealing as a Bostonian longshoreman, and is as handsome as a sack of Irish potatoes," one Chief allegedly said upon hearing the news.

Still, HMCS Wink is not pleased with the results of the award and is asserting his triad executive privilege order a recount of the award.

There are rumors swirling that this will not end well for our stoic First Classes. "Out in the desert, no one can hear you scream," says an Officer with multiple deployments of experience. "Hazing, reprisal and retribution are only recommendations in the jungles of Afghanistan."

Although it may sound silly that anyone would get upset about not being named the unit Leprechaun, this should not diminish the notable achievement of Petty Officer Roberts.

> Imagine a short, Irish fellow who carries gold in his pockets and gives children cavities. Or nightmares, whichever.

Anonymous sources have cited Roberts training for this job since the McGregor Days. He'd talk in his accent while sleeping.

"An outstanding method actor, one we can all aspire to. HM2 Roberts is better than Senior Chief in every way for this award."

OLD-MAN CANDY CAUSES SURGEONS TO FLOCK LIKE CROWS

A murder of doctors have been seen flocking over to the pharmacy more often than normal, and it is being decided as to why.

The leading theory is that there is now an abundance of "old-man" candy in the treat bowl outside of the outpatient pharmacy window.

No one knows for sure how the peppermint lozenges arrived there, but evidence is pointing towards the chaplain having a little bit of fun with the junior folks. No one is laughing from the Surgical Suite though.

"The surgeons and that one anesthesiologist are attracted to this candy how deer are to the salt block," says one bluejacket.

With all the jaw-jacking the surgeons do over their coffees and Metamucil, a little mint or hardened caramel really tie them over until their first naps of the day.

One anesthesiologist swears by the old prune juice and Lifesaver combination to start any day.

"Back when I was getting trucked by Junior Seau, this would set me straight," they allegedly admitted.

SEL GOT NOTHING FOR HM BIRTHDAY, CHIEFS ALWAYS LOSE SHIT OVER NOTHING

Chief AT is upset because he did not get anything for the Hospital Corps Birthday. No one is surprised because Chief always goes crazy over nothing.

Despite being the butt of a terrible joke, Chief was seen visibly distressed when a routing folder was not in the "preferred" font of Times New Roman, and was instead in the old Navy's "Courier New" style.

The offender, no other than HM1 Ellen DeGeneres himself was thought to make the old goat happy by reminding him of the times before Sky Hook.

Chief was of course not impressed with this gesture. Chief supposedly said that the Navy was best when the Officers could beat the Enlisted and you never saw your Chief unless it was at your Captains Mast.

"This is the way of the Anchor," said one all-too-eager First Class, "To make their Sailors feel like they haven't accomplished anything until that EOT award is presented."

We do know that the USN stands for Unity, Service and Navigation though, and should win at least one round at Buffalo Wild Wings Trivia night.

TAKE OFF YOUR HAT IN MEDICAL, YOU LOOK DUMB

> **"Have some respekt for the sick, dying and the dead. Take off your damn hat while in medical"**

Once upon a time when the Camel was just a one hump chump, there he was, stuck on a real Navy warship.

The Camel has been chewed out before, he knows all about getting yelled at, just ask him. Possibly the worst he ever received was when he walked into the medical spaces with his Uncle Joe Camel baseball cap, thinking he was being fashionable. You know, hip, rad and cool.

Chief had other thoughts unfortunately, and the fire and brimstone began to reign down upon the one hump chump.

What makes this story so interesting and worth sharing is that Chief was not a Corpsman. As rude, crude and lewd as he was with his vocabulary, inflection and syntax, the point was made very clearly at a very young age:

Have some respekt for the sick, dying and the dead. Take off your damn hat while in medical.

"But Camel, you're still just a one-hump chump, what do you know about looking cool and hip and rad? Why you treading on me, you snek?," I hear you say.

To clarify, the Camel now has three humps in him at his age, you miserable piece of shit. Secondly, where throwing rocks in glass houses isn't the MO of this publication, the Camel does work with other Sailors who do not take care of themselves and already have sky-rocketed blood pressure. Together we can help save them from themselves.

Don't be judged, be praised, be respected and not seen as an inconsiderate joke. The Camel has your back, all humps.

NURSES BEGGED TO ATTEND "COUNT BY FIVES" WORKSHOP

Nurses in the Intensive Care Unit are begged by their department head to attend the "Count By Fives" workshop held by clinic mascot Sammy in order to get through narcotic turnover at a decent time.

"If they would could count tablets by five instead of two's or each one individually, we wouldn't have the exhaustion excuses I've been hearing lately," bemoaned a clueless bureaucrat.

It is true that time is money, but it is also alertness and empathy. The longer it takes to do a job that literally a two year old in a quasi-permanent helmet can do is a mark of the current state of our Nurse Corps.

The pharmacy staff is also here to help, often playing dual roles of Caregiver Occupational Stress Control (CgOSC) "buddies."

"It ain't much, but it's honest work" says one funny looking pharmacy technician, "nurses cry to use like we are their parole officers, but really we just want to deliver the "Michael Jackson drugs" and go back to the gym.

You hang in there nurses of the ICU. You'll get paid to do nothing like the ED one day soon enough. Until that day, keep your stick on the ice.

Volume I, Issue 4 Page 3

CDR GARDNER BEGINS TRAINING FOR KAF STRONGMAN COMPETITION

The Director of Medical Services is calling his shot on Swole 3, and quite frankly anyone who graces it with their presence.

"First of all, calling it 'Swole 3' is a stupid name. It's called a 'War Gym' and we need to start addressing it as such," the tip of the ED may have stated.

There has been a noticeable uptick in testosterone prescriptions according to the pharmacy staff. By placing the pieces together, The Thirsty Camel is suggesting that CDR Gardner is on 'roid rage benders in preparation for the KAF Strongman Competition being held later this summer.

"From all the YouTube videos he's watching of 'The Mountain' setting the world record in dead lifting, we believe that he is just getting amped up to turn the 'War Gym' inside out," stated an ED LPO.

The amount of whey protein the senior officer is consuming should be concerning, but it is not. Many believe that because he is a doctor who doesn't get upset about anything should rate him excusable for competing against the base's biggest meat heads.

CDR Gardner could not be reached for comment. He was supposedly at the DFAC getting his calories in for the day so that he can sling the iron. We all know anyone in the ED has the sort of time to dedicate to this tall task.

[Generic Strongman meme here]

THE ART OF NAME-CALLING

Whiskey's Patient Administration Department, or PAD to the layman, is in a very unique situation. They are given the distinct job to name all of the patients who get admitted to the Role 3 MMU.

In case anyone has been living under a bridge and closed off from the social world that KAF has to offer, PAD caught a blitz or infamy when they made the unilateral decision to name patients after Star Wars characters. This would not have been as big of a problem had they decided to actually pick good names. Instead, they chose a random combinations of letters and numbers.

Note to future-PAD decision makers, giving our patients the names of fictional droids is puzzling at best and typically frustrating. If PAD wasn't busy letting the shit-sucker-uppers onto the compound, a more serious moment would be taken to explain this.

This is why a clinic petition is being drafted to get away from the barbaric pop culture references where the plague of identity politics precedes quality content and storytelling. If the PAD is going to be funny, it's going to be mandated to root their sense of humor in something that is objectively funny, and not burdened with forced make believe first world issues.

Quality name-calling would exponentially increase should PAD turn their attention to media which forced us to come together as a nation and withstand the test of time.

"They are given the distinct job to name all of the patients who get admitted to the Role 3 MMU"

MASCAS cases come in groups, and we should name our patients as such. The cast of the ThunderCats, Mighty Morphin' Power Rangers, TMNT, or the A-Team are perfectly suitable and appropriate. If Game of Thrones didn't shit the bed the final 3 seasons, they'd have an argument.

EDWARDS AND ROBINSON FIGHT OVER WHO IS NICEST OF THEM ALL

Butterbean "practicing"

How real Americans practice conflict resolution

It's not every day we get to see a good old fashioned hockey fight, but the sticks are being dropped and gloves are coming off in the ICU.

Growing beef between LCDR Edwards and HM2 Robinson has been building over who just is the nicest staffer in the Whiskey unit, and they are going to deal with it as sea warring desert docs do.

The first annual "Drop 'bows, Not ICE Comments" is currently under review and on the XO's desk now.

"We've heard of 'War on the Shore' and 'Rumble in the Jungle,' but KAF is about to experience 'Trial By Combat in Marpat,'" says the amateur promoter, HM2 Jed Rodriguez. By now, meaningful buzz phrases are just part of the job for the moppy-headed Rodriguez. Says Rod, "these promotable evaluations don't write themselves you know."

The buildup to these extravaganza event is causing a ruckus within the ranks. HM2 Arboleda is petitioning the Afghanistan Gaming Commission to apply for his bookie license in order to take legal bets.

Meanwhile, the cage-fighting DCSS Director is busy training and waiting to be unleashed and raise holy Hell across the land.

DRUMHELLER WANTS TO UNCANCEL OKTOBERFEST

Petty Officer Justin Drumheller has maintained a steady diet of Amstel Near Beers, and it's beginning to show. This proud man of German heritage is trying to uphold his part of continuing a proud legacy.

It has come to no surprise then that on one of the latest benders from the barracks, he was heard to say that, "My people won't stand for this, we're uncancelling Oktoberfest for the masses. Martin Luther will be proud of me yet."

This is of course very problematic for military leadership since we are in the trenches of COVID warfare. A follower among the surgical team, Drumheller states that he's ready to step up and lead his people back to the fatherland once his obligation in Afghanistan is up.

Whether or not Drumheller will get what he wants is largely dependent on forces way outside his control. "I want to uncancel the only celebration my countrymen can still offer to the world. Most of the time it's not cool to be German these days, or for the past 70 or so years."

JOHN AND RASTALL AUDITION FOR PRESTIGIOUS DANCE STUDIO

Being a Second Class Petty Officer can feel more like being trapped on Cut Throat Island or in an episode of Game of Thrones (one of the first four seasons). The only place more competitive and sad to travel is through the First Class Mess. That is exactly what it is too, a mess.

Annual evaluations are no joke, and trying to separate yourself from your peers can be a tall order and daunting task. Only the top 20% of those eligible can be recommended for the highest score on an evaluation.

That is why it was it was nearly incredible when two of Whiskey's own auditioned for a sole spot on a prestigious community service dance studio. The studio claims to provide entertainment for more than 50% of the population.

In order to break out from the mold, and create new sources of leadership, quality of work and teamwork, these two Petty Officers gave it their all at the dance audition.

Dancing to Eddie Money's "Take Me Home Tonight" and Billie Eilish's "Bad Guy" the two titans of the floor commenced a fierce dance battle. Calories were torched, palpations occurred, and jazz hands set the stage on fire.

Live from KAF!! Swayze and Farley. Classic skit. Again, copyright.

Two of the Navy's finest dance-off for top spot

"It's all in the spirit of promoting a better Navy," said Rastall, "I think I had the edge for 'the look', but John definitely edged me out in spirit animal energy. I couldn't be more proud to go to war than with this guy."

HM2 John agrees saying, "No matter who wins, I know that I gave my best and was tried against the best. It's really going to help me grow knowing that I was with the biggest of giants."

Both Sailors agree that promotion of the Navy is the number one motivating factor for trying out for this position. They also agree that the quality of life if best when politics are left at the door and you simply try to make each day your masterpiece.

The Whiskey brass is applauding these two's burning desire to try new things. Says one Okie reservist officer, "if I was 25 years younger I would be out there joining them."

Competition breeds the best in any market and these two are fighting tooth and nail to best serve the Navy while promoting a healthy lifestyle.

From all perspectives, the decided winner is too close to call. The announcement will come later next week.

JESSE JOHN

Conventional wisdom states to never trust a man with two first names. There was nothing conventional about my friendship with HM2 (FMF) Jesse John. Of all the people I met in Whiskey, I considered Jesse my best friend. There were people I spoke to more, who I had more impactful encounters with and saw more frequently, but Jesse was different.

He was the Stern to my Oskar, the Teller to my Penn. When I was being bombastic and full of charisma, he held back and was reserved. I always found myself gravitating to people who I aspire to be like, and with that belief there is a very natural tendency to stick closely to a guy like Jesse. There are two kinds of people, the "guy" and the "guy who the guy depends on." Jesse didn't say much, he didn't have to. What we shared was, I think, a completion of the other half.

We took turns earning each other's trust. I think I was more willing to give it than he was, but it was an honor when we'd kick back, just him and I, to talk about things. Where we came from, how it made us to what we are, and where we see ourselves going. He was an admirable reader, and it was a privilege to know why. He was athletic while I was jolly. He was a good sport around me, and I tried to reciprocate that too.

Although most stories between us will sink to the bottom of Davy Jones' locker before I would release them to the world, upholding an oath to honorably keep what he shared with me private, they are still something to be cherished. Who knows the complete story of Jesse John? Certainly not me, our time was too short, but what I did come to learn will stick with me, and it was my pleasure to get to know him how I did.

23 Jun 20
Day 126 & 127

Talk about the two most bleak days of the deployment so far. Today I was sleeping and most of yesterday was sleeping too.

June 22 we had a diversity committee meeting. All went well and according to schedule until we got to the point of discussing what we wanted to do for July. I suppose in a way it came naturally, but if I were to listen to myself, I would have thought that I hijacked the meeting. Essentially, I used my connections as a PAO member to infuse the agenda of diversity into the newsletter. I mentioned something about it to HM1 Wilson how I felt along those lines, and he said that he liked what I did. Now I just need to produce, again.

One might say that COVID precautions are beginning to really pick up. LCDR Deguzman said that unless we really have a reason to be at work then do not be in the pharmacy. This is actually going to be really hard as I am finding out.

I still left work after lunch and went home to go to bed. I slept until dinner. Drumheller is very particular about going to chow between 1700-1730. I pushed it to 1730, and I popped 75 mg of Benadryl and went to sleep. I didn't wake up until 0830 the next day. I really surprised myself.

I'm beginning to wonder what is keeping me from reading Stephen King's *Dr. Sleep* because I'm jumping to Netflix when I get the chance. I'm still working on Steve Carrell's *Space Force* (2020) and Bill Burr's *F is for Family* (2015). One resource I did discover today, although I heard about it weeks ago was KAF.TV. They have many movies and television shows to explore.

Because I had gotten tired enough to do something about it, and I wanted to engage HM1 LaPenna in a heated debate, my curious mind finally watched *The Goonies.* Truth be told, I was not impressed. To me, it was a group of friends who wandered deeper into a convenient tunnel and were saved at the last minute at every moment of danger. I'll really have to ask what the big deal is because I definitely did not get it.

I slept through breakfast and took another nap through lunch so by dinner I was beginning to get hungry. Before that, I called the boys. Josiah had swimming lessons, so he was especially tired. Atticus was causing mischief, again, but was looking cute doing it so it cancels out. Saori is busy trying to stand up her new website design and I can tell she's getting nervous because she's asking me many questions. Some I can answer, but others are her decision. I just have to do a better job supporting her, I think.

Anyway, I couldn't sleep so I walked into work early and began writing.

Postscript: Some people only did the job of their billet during the deployment. Others went above and beyond the call of duty and bounced from this committee to that committee. For the most part, both were evaluated appropriately for it. I think I was part of the latter group, but it never caused me to stop thinking about how different my life in Afghanistan would have been had I stuck to the bare minimum. What if I focused only on me when I wasn't immediately helping the mission? Would I have gone to the gym more? Would I have experienced burnout? How might I have been here? Would I have had anything to particularly write about? Did I choose the path not taken, and did it make all the difference? Even now I still wonder about these questions.

26 Jun 20
Days 128, 129 & 130

Is this what my days are turning into, one entry every three days? I hope not, but if there is one recurring theme lately it's that I need to get more disciplined. There isn't one specific thing either, but a collection of many different aspects of my life.

I think one of the biggest changes is that I'm collecting boxes and beginning to start shipping things back. There are things I have definitely not used, nor intend to while I'm here. I have over-packed and it's time to ship it back. Little by little though. My thought is that when I come back it will be there in Japan. I'm not ready to mail a majority of my books back, but clothes and maybe some toiletries.

Today we did not have any patients. Our one patient, the general, was transferred back to the host nation hospital yesterday in order for his family to give their final goodbyes. That was tough, the guy also did not make it easy for me. Every time he crashed, it seemed like it was on my shift. I had to learn a lot about inpatient pharmacy from this guy. Obviously he didn't know that, nor did he care, but in his passing he helped me become a stronger pharmacy technician.

Because we do not have a patient, the decision was made to start our workday at 0900. I think this should excite me, but it doesn't. Starting the day at that time is too late. By then it's starting to get too hot to walk, breakfast is cold, or not even available, and I'm too conditioned to get rolling earlier. I'll possibly become conditioned to accept the change, but I'm going to try and hold out for as long as possible.

Speaking of holding out, Issue #5 of *The Thirsty Camel* is complete. What I want to do is wait until July 1, I've already made four issues in June alone. Pretty sure though we have been in the same situation before, and my excitement will not be able to be contained. I'll remain optimistic though, and I'll grow some self-discipline.

The command climate survey is done and LCDR Deguzman is building the report for it. Rumor has it the CO isn't happy with the results, but LCDR is actually satisfied. Not totally sure where this disparity comes from, but it does not diminish the fact that I really would have liked to be on the command climate team, or "resilience" team, so that I can look at the problem more closely.

Oh well, here is a crumb of good news, I manscaped today! It's very exciting news to me. While Drumheller was at work, I did the deed. Since I didn't know exactly when he'd be home, it was a bit of a rush job, but I made it work. My chest hair no longer sticks out from my shirt.

My sleep schedule is quite screwy, and I don't like it. I wish I could stick to a basic plan, but life and circumstances get in the way. I think this goes back to being in my head way too much.

I had a really nice talk with HM1 LaPenna. There is something about smoke deck confessionals that I just love. It was just he and I out there, talking, but this talk had a bit more of a purpose. If it were totally simplified, I think it could be chalked up as "help me help you." I might be the Second Class, but my head is in the mindset that I need to perform as a First. He's not totally great about some things that I enjoy doing, but I want to offer my help because that's what good teammates do. In the meantime, I am off doing my own thing, but I'm also here for the team.

I did however make him teach me how to read the recipe book one more time more thoroughly. I believe I'm more comfortable, but not solid, about the medications though. This takes time and as mentioned before, the best prescription is getting repetitions.

Of course, the boys were just as lovely and beautiful when I called. Miss them a lot.

Postscript: This is a very telling entry. I was able to explain a lot that was going on both for myself and those around me. Should I do this deployment over again, and knowing what I do now, I know that I would mail a lot less crap. Some staff packed more than I did, and I had boxes and boxes of stuff. Why would I need to mail two fans? Why would I need all those civilian clothes? We had to either be in our Army uniform, or "OCP," our Navy Physical Training Uniform (PTU), or a command authorized shirt. I brought along way too many books, but I was anticipating putting in my time at the pharmacy, going back to my room, and being a monk. That didn't happen. HM1 LaPenna was so interesting to me. It took a lot for him to have a bad day, was the best pound-for-pound technician I ever met, and it took a lot for him to let me know when his buttons were pushed. Of course, when I was able to do that, as I have clearly established a knack for with people I absolutely shouldn't, he let me know, which made me feel worse.

Editor's Note: The back-to-back Camel *issues are not a mistake. Issue #5 was released on 27 June 2020 and Issue #6 was shown to the world on 6 July 2020.*

Definitely Not a NATO Role 3 MMU Publication

The Thirsty Camel

Volume 1, Issue 5

Published Gandalf style: Exactly when it was meant to arrive.

Special points of interest:

- Australians do not have sex. Australians mate.
- Texting is the way to mis-communicate how you feel, and misinterpret what other people mean.
- CAPT Klinger has picked up the collateral of Whiskey Librarian.
- Why doesn't America tell knock-knock jokes? Because Freedom Rings.
- HM2 Roberts is an accent away from being Joe Pesci.

Inside this issue:

Moonlight Doc	2
Navy's Father	2
Coke "Lite"	2
Croc Dundee	3
Inside Story	3
'MURICA!	3
Nickelback	4

UNCLE SAM SADDLES UP FOR USO TOUR

American mascot Uncle Sam is getting arrangements in order to conduct yet another 4th of July USO Tour for the troops.

Although Uncle Sam is seen at most post offices, recruitment centers and other hubs of propaganda, this tour is particularly important to the two-time World War Champion.

"I just like seeing the men and women who have to suffer through deployments. Even Whiskey with their air-conditioning, paved roads, toilet closets, and beds need a little encouragement from time to time, and this is the day of the year to let them know they aren't forgotten," says Uncle Sam at a phone interview with the Thirsty Camel.

Uncle Sam wanted the rest of the deployed folks out there to know that even though he's got the sciatica , he's still going to be marching and PT-ing with them bright and early.

"Leadership leads from the front, and that's where I intend to be. Kick ass and chew bubble gum got Rowdy Roddy Piper a second career, and it will get you through these tough times."

Uncle Sam has certainly been busy in recent months, doing what he can to kick the COVID-19's ass and looking for a vaccine.

"I really want Whiskey to make it to Sembach, Germany for multiple reasons. First and foremost, there is beer there, and a lot of it. Nothing breaks tension, builds longer tables and breaks more walls more than a cold "Steveweiser."

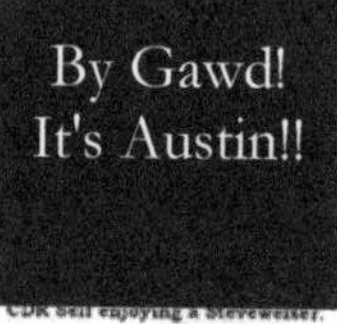

CDR Sell enjoying a Steveweiser.

Uncle Sam telling you to be concerned w/ copyright

Uncle Sam kicks ass and chews bubble gum. And he's all out of bubble gum.

Uncle Sam will storm the beaches, he will pick up arms, he will never forget where we as Americans came from. He wishes to close with following remarks:

"We will not go quietly into the night!

We will not vanish without a fight!

We're going to live on!

We're going to survive!"

KAF 3 ON 3 LINE-UPS DUE

In the case that anyone actually takes this publication seriously, the 3-on-3 basketball deadline is fast approaching for the Independence Day show-down.

Pictured here is General George Washington posterizing Kim Jung-un while Abraham Lincoln boxes out Comrade Joseph Stalin. Not pictured at the top the key was Theodore Roosevelt.

Up to four players can be on a team. Thomas Jefferson was busy flirting with the cheerleaders, but was more than ready to break ankles.

Team Rushmore is thrilled to compete against KAF's finest.

George Washington posterizing Kim Jong-Un while Lincoln boxes out Stalin

CDR NASH MOONLIGHTS AS RENT-A-DAD

Not a stock photo of a rent-a-dad, move along

Commander Judd Nash recently sat down with the Thirsty Camel to discuss a growing market and one he is very excited about exploring.

He has discovered that there is a need for the rent-a-dad career. Although still an anesthesiologist and Navy Reservist, he feels this is the best way to pay off for his kids' education and meet new people.

"All the people I meet at my day job are either asleep or about to be zonked out," says the Colorado resident, "This is a great way to feel relevant and needed again. My kids are teenagers now and too cool for their old man."

The rent-a-dad profession is quite simple: college students who attend university far from home still want to have the old man around, at barbecue's especially , but only on their terms.

CDR Nash laughs, "really they just want me to come over with my grill and I whip something up and tell them stories. They tip big time when I call them "sport," "big guy," "champ," or "shooter."

By tipping "big time" CDR is actually referring to an unlimited access to the beer cooler. After months choking down the Near Beers at KAF, an old fashioned barley pop is actually just what the doctor ordered, no pun intended.

"This job would not have been possible without the concurrent invention of services such as Lyft and Uber," Dr. Nash explains, "because it can be really difficult getting home after getting totally loaded."

After hearing of the emerging field, Whiskey's Executive Officer is also interested in this gig.

"I'm really close to retirement and will need a new hobby to get out of the house," says Whiskey's #2.

Not a job for everyone, and certainly not for the self-admitted cheap date either.

"We are a fighting force which prides itself from separating Church and State."

JOHN PAUL JONES NO LONGER YOUR DADDY

Top Navy executives are jumping on the latest fad of removing its most famous leaders of the past from the books.

John Paul Jones will henceforth no longer be considered the father of the Navy according to a recent publication coming from the Pentagon.

"John Paul is a name too close to Pope John Paul II, and we are a fighting force which prides itself from separating Church and State," reasoned one top brass Sailor.

The publication went on to reassure the Chaplain Corps that there was still a place for them among the deckplates. The Dental Corps is not pleased though with the decision.

One Naval dentist, "Eighty-percent of Chap's job is walking around jaw-jacking and passing out all that sugary candy. It's making us actually have to work, and we can't have that. Why even go to dental school?"

The nuclear community originally had their concerns about Admiral Rickover's place as the father of the nuclear Navy, but were quickly put at ease.

"Anyone that crotchety yet genius at the same time could be anyone's old man somewhere."

FREDDIE OFFERS FAIR BUT FIRM OFFER

COKE LITE

Supply Warehouse technician Freddie is so nice he makes Mr. Rogers look like an asshole. His office is like a confession booth when Chaps is out. He's patient, wise and respectful.

The staff at the Thirsty Camel wants to be clear, like crystal, Freddie could probably kick the Hulk's ass should he ever feel inclined to do so.

It is this balance that makes the following story so sensational. The other day, an editor for The Thirsty Camel was supporting his director and acquiring more Coke "Lite's" than he really needed.

Let it be known that Freddie also enjoys his daily ration of Coke Lite. When it was observed the kitchen raider in question was being more of a capitalist than a socialist, the prior Army Captain fired off a warning shot that shown high and bright.

Due to space concerns, the alleged conversation is paraphrased to Freddie promising to ensure a new hump was formed on the Thirsty Camel after he inserted his fist far enough through his face to create one. Lesson here: don't hoard. Here's another lesson for the savages: It's called Diet Coke, not Coke Lite.

HOW MOLLAH GOT HIS ARKANSAS TOOTHPICK

He has many names, but if we were to ask where Crocodile Dundee worked, we would resoundingly retort that he could be found in the Emergency Department.

What exactly Specialist Mollah is doing in the ED could be anyone's guess, and even if "nothing" is a very practical prediction, we ought to take pause and reflect to not only his contribution to Role 3's mission, but also just where he acquired the Jackhawk 9000 knife he is renown for.

Rumor has it Mollah came across his knife after watching another movie in the ED called, "Talladega Nights: the legend of Ricky Bobby." There Ricky Bobby was sponsoring the Rambo blade for sale at Wal-Mart. Thinking it was a joke, the junior enlisted solider headed over to his nearest Baron of Capitalism and sure enough, it was in stock.

That is the "official" story. The Camel brings the facts though. Mollah got that blade from a local Afghanistan native. The local was in need of shipping some local "flowers" out of the country. Although the details are murky, and the translation loose, there was something to be said about competition, turf wars, and Columbia.

Just an advertisement of Ricky Bobby trying to sell the Jackhawk 9000 knife to any ignorant soul. Ah whatever, don't have the license for this pic either.

The emergency department is fortunate to have Crocodile Dundee for as long as NCIS remains clueless and in the dark.

"Hi, I'm Ricky Bobby, and if you don't chew Big Red, then f*ck you."

130 AND COUNTING...

If anyone should ever wonder why the Role 1 Army medics and officers are seemingly the most miserable lot of the whole damn bunch put together, the Camel is here with the scoop.

On the board behind the Role 1 desk is a number. At the time of this article, the number stands at 130. This number is the consecutive days the Army has reported for duty.

Unlike the Navy, the Army seemingly enjoys beating the holy Hell out of their manpower until they are as happy as we see them these days.

Role 3 staff should take note at the level of dedication the Army is bringing to the mission. Like a dedicated father who sold his dreams down the river so that he could provide for their family, Role 1 carries a "workin' man blues" swagger to their step, but they are up and at it every single day.

"If our technicians had a fraction of the grit that Role 1 drags in every day, maybe things would be different," says one cage-fighting director, "I'm not even going to comment on the nurses."

It doesn't matter if they see 1 patient or 100 per day, they are there, present, each and every day. It sort of makes a cocky camel rethink about some things.

"If our technicians had a fraction of the grit that Role 1 drags in every day, maybe things would be different"

LEST WE FORGET HOW AWESOME AMERICA TRULY IS

By now, we should collectively come to the conclusion that the staff here at the Thirsty Camel is very proud to be American. In fact, Little Camel's are born on the 4th of July, and you can fact check that, Politico.

We might be working, we may have "the day off," but Whiskey will still be here, together, in sunny Afghanistan. The Camel is glad he's stuck here with everyone, no matter what they try to tell you around the watercooler.

To claim that we are American and in this same foxhole together reminds me that what we are doing is something incredibly special.

Take notes because this moment of serenity is not supposed to be here. Laugh at the bad jokes, share what we have, and enjoy the days we have together. We are not perfect, we are human, and it's that spice of life which makes this all worth while. Try, help, and one day this war will end. Anyway, it's a real pleasure writing for you all.

Teddy Roosevelt laying down lead against the sasquatch at the Battle of the Bulge. Trust me, I got it from the Internet.

America being AWESOME

Volume 1, Issue 5 Page 3

George Washington carried by a bald eagle with an American flag in its talons with a rocket launcher.

Ronald Reagan on a velociraptor with an Uzi fighting off commies as Old Glory flaps proudly in the back.

Ron Swanson, a true American, with an American flag flapping in the foreground. Quote by HM1 LaPenna, "I write because I want to, not because I care."

Abraham Lincoln with what appears to be the Gettysburg Address in one hand and M16 in the other hand. While mounted on a grizzly bear to complete the America As F@#k series of portraits.

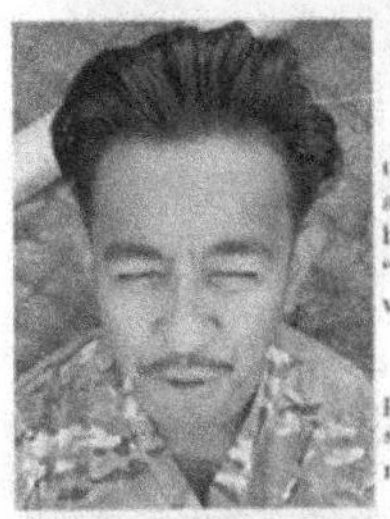

Chad Kroeger circa 2007.

Rodriguez is the Whiskey Nickelback

Here is a little thought experiment, the next time you are feeling bad about yourself, know that you could have been named the unit's "Nickelback." That is the case for our very own HM2 Jed Rodriguez.

Let's examine the facts and compare. The most glaring, undisputable similarity is the desperate need to rethink hairstyle.

Our second point to mention is the pathetic utilization of facial hair. If the Department of the Navy authorized hair to grow on our chinny chin chins, HM2 Rodriguez would attempt to look just as embarrassing. In fairness, points to the good HM2 for giving it the old college try with what he has though.

Third, like Nickelback, HM2 is comic relief even when it is absolutely unintentional. He really is the king with this, much like Canada's national treasure.

Like Nickelback, HM2 Rodriguez is excellent company for all occasions. He is diverse, can rock, but also spit out some rather profound poetry with that silver tongue of his.

Petty Officer Rodriguez can offer words of encouragement too, just like the band. He has this instinct of drawing you in, leading you no choice but to listen to his message.

Nickelback has a terrible reputation, but like an ogre, has layers of complexity. Rod is no different, some might think he does nothing except smoke, play video games and lift, but he's actually the biggest cheerleader in multiple shipmate's corners. Don't look now, but he might actually be enjoyable to have around.

The lead singer for Nickelback, Chad Kroeger was able to marry Avril Lavigne in her prime, so that is a leg-up for Team Canada, but Rod is still on his first marriage. In today's climate and military culture, a true mark of stability and extraordinary patience.

We seriously doubt anyone in Nickelback could lay claim to being part of the 1000lb club either, but they're big rock stars. They have guitars, Rod just makes everyone feel good calling them "king".

Indeed, HM2 Rodriguez should be proud to be Whiskey's Nickelback, even if we can all take turns making fun of him for such a high honor. He reminds us who we really are.

Special points of interest:

- If women don't find you handsome, they should at least find you handy.
- Krombach's memoir, "The time I walked from the barracks into work," categorized as fiction
- Imagine a world where we loved each other as much as LCDR Salazar loves the N95.
- HM1 LaPonna asks more useless questions than Plato and Socrates should they have a love-child

Volume I , Issue VI

Published: Who cares, just enjoy the wasted time some people take to make you people laugh.

The Thirsty Camel

Definitely not a NATO Role 3 Publication

CAMEL'S BACK. BACK AGAIN. CAMEL'S BACK. TELL A FRIEND.

After a brief hiatus to see what else there is to do, the Camel has decided that there isn't much fun without making fun of all of you.

So it's been awhile and out of the game, and you thought the Camel got lame. No one should care who's writing this bit, just something to laugh at while you're taking your sh*t.

What really chaps his ass is he's told he's lost his bit, but he's just reloading for the next greatest hit.

Gather round and hear the Great One speak, he be clapping bad rhymes until you all weak.

PAD, Surgeons and nurses too, the stories write themselves, he'd make fun of the lab, but they're all smoking in the back room.

To our Officers bless their hearts, we know it's you exploding the male bathroom upstairs with your farts. You all try your best, but good thing they don't have to worry about passing any test.

Of leadership that is because they are too busy clawing for that extra day off, it's embarrassing, you should be enlisted and then try to answer the call.

Superman "S" shield. Because the "S" means hope, supposedly.

Whiskey is weird and there is no doubt, when lieutenants share rooms it's exactly how contempt comes about.

For all of you who think the Camel's lost his step, just flip through these pages and see what he's got left.

He's not the hero we deserve, but the one we need, to keep our sanity together, just to spot the obvious and plant the seed.

It was all a dream, never did it ever occur that being creative would pick up so much steam. But you kept laughing so the Camel kept writing, watching it grow has been a bit enlightening.

So no more carved flags in the head. Manny would not appreciate that, show off your pride without cowardice instead.

Be good or be bad, come skeptical, leave glad. Chase the buck, but above all else you must remember to not suck.

Soon this will be all over and maybe even thought of as a joke, only a few more lines, almost time for another Diet Coke.

Again I'll say it again, and as loud as I can, the Camel is back so tell a friend. If he's ever doubted and questioned again, consider yourself persona non grata, you'll make the next front page news and this is where the article ends.

WILSON BEATS KUBIL IN B-BALL, CONVINCED IS GOD'S GIFT

HM1 Jacob Wilson has managed to defeat Whiskey basketball stand-out HM1 Jake Kubil in a couple of consecutive games of one-on-one.

As a result, HM1 Wilson has not shut up about his heroic triumph, being heard to say that two back-to-back wins makes a streak.

The rare feat has the DCSS LPO convinced that he has been anointed as God's gift to not only the court, but to the Navy too.

Unfortunately being named after a volleyball is not the last cruel joke that was played on Wilson. Over the course of the next six games, he was out worked, out hustled and outplayed by the Lilliputian Kubil.

Yes, if Tyson ever boxed Mayweather, one well-landed punch would send the tiny man into another universe, but speed kills and Tyson would have to eventually try and catch the pound for pound better player.

Inside this issue:

Trident Bound	2
Davey's Still in the Navy	2
CIO's Cookies	2
DCSS in Hot seat	3
ICU Nurses Learned	3
Motivational Speaker	3
Where's my boy Vinnie Chase?!	4

HM2 JOHN IS NOT BUD/S DUD, QUIT ASKING

With so many people in this world being strung up for stolen valor, it is important for the Thirsty Camel to do the ethically right thing to do and assist a staff member within the Whiskey Rotation.

By no means has HM2 John ever been a Navy SEAL, and he has never claimed to be one. There is a mountain of evidence which may suggest a different story, but the Camel is here to set the facts straight and dispel any rumors.

Although Petty Officer John has the haircut which aligns with someone who has might have graced the Coronado beaches, that does not mean he is, was, or ever wanted to be a Frogman.

His peculiar familiarity with firearms and weapons of considerable destruction is a fluke coincidence. He was a traditionally-trained firearms instructor while with the Marines.

Trident

He's fit, like disproportionally fit compared to his ranked peers. He looks like Brad Pitt, but not the "Troy" Brad Pitt, the Tyler Durden flavor of bringing sexy back. If you cared about your body enough, you'd put in the effort too. Senior Chief tries, but he has constant "back pain" to finish sculpting the lower half of his body.

HM2 John can't even spell BUD/S, and it's doubtful he can spell DUD either, but that's the beauty of him because he's always reading in his spare time.

With a Sailor who keeps his story so close to his chest, John is actually a remarkable shipmate and Corpsman. Whiskey is lucky to be able to call him our own.

He doesn't prove it by jaw-jacking his way to the top of any list, board, or collateral. He proves it through his actions and willingness to fail when so many are apt to pull back in fear of the unknown consequence.

So maybe he is like a SEAL, but who knows, the Camel can only speculate.

DAVEY IS STILL IN THE NAVY, AND IS SALTY ABOUT IT

"Davey Jones is a [expletive] legend, and we can't let any of our history leave at this time. If Seaman Timmy can't leave, neither can Davey."

The highly prolific Sailor in Billy Joel's anthem "Piano Man" is in fact still in the Navy despite his many attempts to archive his career, the Department of the Navy resists.

Known to all as simply "Davey," David Jones has sailed around the world many times over, and is said to even sleep at the bottom of the ocean.

"Davey Jones is a [expletive] legend, and we can't let any of our history leave at this time. If Seaman Timmy can't leave, neither can Davey," stated a Command Senior Enlisted Advisor.

Indeed, Davey is still in the Navy, and it looks like he will be entombed beneath the waves of Neptune for life.

Not all is lost however. The Salty Jones has started many a tradition within the maritime force such as be the inspiration of a couple of mildly popular Johnny Depp films and have an honorable mention in the official Navy fight song, "Anchors Aweigh."

Billy Joel was just a man at his piano, but if he knows Davey Jones, then you should too.

NO OATMEAL RAISIN COOKIES, CIO DOES BEST BOBBY KNIGHT IMPERSONATION

With great power comes great responsibility. That is the running gag throughout the ranks in our Navy, but Whiskey Chief Information Officer Lieutenant Eric Porter never got the memo.

In a fit of blinding rage, LT Porter embarked on a tantrum last seen by former Indiana basketball coach Bobby Knight when he threw a chair across the Role 3 galley.

The moment that sparked the outcry was allegedly the duty crew had the chance to grab more Oatmeal Raisin Cookies from the Monti DFAC, but deferred.

"CIO was visibly in a mood today because the oatmeal and raisins are good supplements for green roughage in order to conduct a proper morning routine," says one credentialed provider.

Picture of Coach Knight throwing chairs across the court.

Reenactment of the events in Role 3 Galley

No apology is scheduled to happen, but Internet might be shut off soon.

DCSS SHOWS PICTURE OF PUNCHING BAG, ORDERED TO XO OFFICE

Afghanistan drug kingpin LCDR Vince Deguzman found himself in the Executive Officer's crosshairs and in his hot-seat the other day after a complaint of a Sailor being threatened with their life.

The latest findings from Thirsty Camel staff discovered that the selected Commander allegedly showed a photograph of his punching bag to a junior enlisted Sailor.

"What we are allowed to disclose is the Sailor, who wishes to remain unnamed, compared the photograph to a father showing off his gun collection to a prospective suitor of his daughter," said Public Affairs Officer LCDR Kathleen Fitzgerald.

The matter is taken very seriously as the new age of Sailors no longer has an ability to take a joke. A more professional Navy means a leaner, more capitalistic minded fighting force. What happens is an unprecedented fallout of grit amongst the ranks and in a time of our "information age," more dumb people.

Google search "Filipino cage fighter" and you have the original image here.

LCDR Vince Deguzman, Director of Clinical Support Services, poses in an undated photograph.

There is substantiated rumors of CDR(sel) Deguzman's history of being a vicious killer in the cage. Reports from a Philippine source strongly suggests that the now-pharmacist has no less than four kills during in-ring action.

"No one is telling the director what to do," Fitzgerald went on in her statement, "we just want to try to tame the tiger before he actually does get out of the cage. His trip to the XO's office was nothing more than a professional formality."

In other reports gathered, it has been heard that LCDR Deguzman once said the perfect process improvement would be " for him to rearrange [your] f*ucking face" to another high profile member of Whiskey rotation, but confirmation on the report could not be made.

LT Warner is reaching out to DCSS in an effort to 'AA' through the possible 'roid rage connections. He had similar outbursts while playing as walk-on at Texas Christian.

ICU NURSES IN-SERVICE TRAINING NEARING COMPLETION

"With so many smart people packed in to one department, there are a lot of dumb administrative hiccups to work through."

In part of an on-going process improvement initiative, the nurses assigned to the Intensive Care Unit have been working towards scanning orders in the correct position to the pharmacy.

Says one enlisted Sailor close to the source, "when we started this initiative, many nurses where not even close to being competent, but bless their hearts they are really giving it an honest effort...some of them at least."

Some of the staff feels patronized for having to be walked through a task so simple, but that is a common misconception.

"With so many smart people packed in to one department, there are a lot of dumb administrative hiccups to work through."

Blanket generalizations are a terrible way to consider a diverse group in any organization, and some believe this constant inconsideration is stemming from the war between the two work-centers.

"When pharmacy stops treating us like crap we will start thinking about putting in the two extra seconds to scan our orders the right way," says an insider close to the story.

PRAKASH HIRES MOTIVATIONAL SPEAKER, BUT CANCELS; DRUMHELLER RISES TO OCCASSION

Commander Prakash tried to get Whiskey back on track after many days off from intense patient care by reaching out to semi-professional basketball legend Jackie Moon of the Flint Tropics.

Unfortunately Mr. Moon had a scheduling conflict with his nose and mound of Columbian bam-bam causing him to abruptly cancel the talk.

In a pinch, the good Officer slapped a wig on surgical technologist HM2 Justin Drumheller to stand in Jackie Moon's place.

The honest effort by the blindsided Drumheller earned him a firm handshake from the Assistant Deputy to the Assistant of All Things Imaginary HM2 Terrell.

No autographs were available for fans at the time of the talk.

He really did look like Jackie Moon to me. Google it.

Drumheller acting as Jackie Moon Of the Flint Tropics

DO YOU HAVE WHAT IT TAKES?

THE STAFF AT THE THIRSTY CAMEL IS PASSING OUT THE OFFICIAL CHALLENGE. IF YOU FEEL THAT YOU CAN BE FUNNY, OR HAVE ALWAYS WANTED TO GET SOMETHING OFF YOUR CHEST, THEN YOU ARE CORDIALLY INVITED TO POST YOUR OWN ARTICLE(S). THAT'S RIGHT, THE CAMEL IS LOOKING TO EXPAND THE EDITORIAL STAFF. THE ONLY REQUIREMENTS ARE TO HAVE A FUNNY TAKE AND NOT TO ABSOLUTELY SUCK! INQUIRE WITH ANY CURRENT WRITER OF THE CAMEL FOR MORE DETAILS.

WHISKEY HELPS, DUH

HM2 SLAGLE IS A WEAPONIZED ARI GOLD

He's feisty, he's short, he's a borderline angry lunatic, but HM2 Slagle gets results and the job done.

Recent polling completed by the Thirsty Camel had identified HM2 Nicholas Slagle as a weaponized Ari Gold. Who is this Gold man? Ari Gold is the super agent on the hit television show "Entourage." What is this hit television show you say? Think "Sex and the City," but for bros.

Ari's most famous quality is his unrelenting loyalty to his boy, and favorite client Vinnie Chase. Here at Whiskey, all of PAD TOC's lambs are little Vinnie Chase's in the eyes of it's watchful shepherd, and mustached hero, one HM2 Slagle.

It doesn't matter who you are or where you sit at the table, if you mess with one of the crew, you're dealing with the wrath of

> Ari Gold, no better friend, no worse enemy. Much like Nick Slagle.

Want to hug it out?

an angry, loyal, defensive Super Petty Officer.

A defector from the Oompa Loompa clan in the East Adirondacks, Petty Officer Slagle and his mustache, David Pretzel, have clung onto a few basic nuggets as to what a leader is. The first is that once and again he likes to show the crew that he is in fact human, as loosely as the term will allow.

The second is the Captain America / Steve Rogers mentality that he can go all day in the defense of those who he cares about. Although it's impossible to like everyone the same, it is clear that he genuinely loves each and every one of the staff in PAD TOC.

As expected, the reciprocated result of his efforts has produced a well-oiled machine that has allowed his team to feel safe and trust their fearless leader.

Some jobs are harder than others, but Slagle will mold even the biggest dumpster fires such as HM3 Alden into pearls of shining examples for anyone to follow.

7 July 2020
Days 131, 132, 133, 134, 135, 136, 137, 138, 139, 140 & 141

Hello journal, remember me? It's your friend, Cal. You know, the guy who wanted to dedicate a page a day to recording his travels, feelings, and thoughts for each day of the deployment that Uncle Sam sent him on. You know, that time spent away from his family, wife, kids, and everything he knows and loves. You know, that project he set out to do no matter what?

Remember when Dr. Chris Rock back in Sasebo told you about medical school and what that experience was like for him? He compared it to eating two pancakes every day. Whether you wanted them or not, they were coming each and every day. In order to finish medical school, you had to eat your pancakes. If you skipped a day, you had four to eat and two more were coming the next day.

You get it, and of course you remember, so what is the major malfunction? I know you aren't terribly busy, and no matter what, you have a page of work cut out in front of you. Now look at you, there are 10 whole pages to make up for it. Will you do it?

Can you fulfill the promise you made to yourself, to those after you who want to know your story? Are you going to renege now, or are you weak and feeling sorry for yourself? Only now we shall see.

Let's begin with what a typical day looks like. I would say boring, but that's too easy of a word. I'm constantly stimulated with thought and action, except that all of these thoughts and actions are mindless moments. They are routine, and they do not easily separate themselves from one day to the next.

In fact, my days are chunked into groups of three days. Day one might begin with my 24-hour shift. Since the general was transferred out, we have been treating the hospital as if there are no inpatients. Well, this is not entirely accurate. Our patient load is minimal, but it got a little crazy over Independence Day, which I will get to a little later.

HM1 Wilson does not like waking up early so he changed the start time from 0800 (the start time that Victor Rotation set) to 0830, and now we are at 0900. I can't say I'm absolutely against it, but I would like to start a little earlier. If I have a long night, which did happen within this stretch of time, it makes for a long few hours until relief comes. What is unique about being here and doing what I do is the minimal separation from one day to the next. On my 24-hour shift, I'm working, doing pharmacy work. HM1 LaPenna is working with me for most of the day because he is a borderline workaholic with less hobbies than body mass.

I've gotten used to calling HM1 Wilson and HM1 LaPenna "Ying and Yang." They are opposites, but they make the whole. Until the day we depart from here, I will never tire of trying to chase LaPenna's hustle and Wilson's methodology. Both are so interesting to emulate and study, and both to me represent what is desirable in a Sailor. There is the better technician and the better Petty Officer. Neither are wrong, and of course there is a gray sliver to the venn diagram.

That brings me to LCDR Deguzman. As time here is dragging along, I like him more and more. He has, to me, become more personable. Unlike LCDR Ihlenfeld who stayed on one side of a line of the officer/enlisted divide, LCDR is a mustang himself. He speaks to us candidly and is approachable. When we first started here, I thought of him as overwhelming, and his cadence of questions was too fast for my ability to process all the information being thrown my way. As time would go on to show, I stuck it out, remained coachable and resilient. It has proven dividends. I am very proud of overcoming these challenges.

The other day we had Sailor of the Month boards. For reasons I still do not know, I was kept from being nominated. Instead, I was a board member for the Junior Sailor of the Month. It was weird because I feel the other board members were the rest of the "A" team, the heavy hitters who I think are the biggest movers and shakers amongst the Second Classes.

Anyway, being on the board just reminded me why I don't like nor appreciate the recognition board process. There was more than one instance that a nominee paid the price for a LPO's misgivings and mistakes. It really made me wonder if I was ever in that situation. I'm sure I had to be with the perception I carried of some of my previous leaders. Looking back on it, I do not blame them, they were human after all, as I am.

To that end, it helped solidify the belief that there is so much more to being a leader than the poor bastard who carries out Chief's wishes. One day I really hope to carry that burden.

There was a new Commanding Officer in Yokosuka and consequently, Sasebo is included. Naturally when this happens there is a command climate survey. Because Sasebo's Officer in Charge, CDR Kyle Dohm, offered a 24-hour special liberty if the clinic reached 90% completion, I offered to do my part and filled it out. What came out surprised me. [The rest of this paragraph has been redacted from the electronic edition until I am at least no longer serving in an active duty status.]

Still on the subject of Sasebo, I emailed Master Chief Lorenzo Branch tonight seeking his opinion on what I ought to do in regard to a MAP, or Meritorious Advancement Program. Essentially, I stated that I know HM2 Yani Lopez was asked again to submit a write-up, and it's her third time being approached by leadership to do so. Was there an "out of sight, out of mind" occurrence, or is there something else I'm overlooking? I know that technically nothing stops me from submitting my name for consideration, but if I was not invited on purpose, that is a bit different than forgetting I exist. The worst thing I can hear is a line of fluff, a cookie cutter answer that will not actually serve any purpose beside leaving me still without guidance.

I'm still working on that Stephen King book. Currently I'm about 200 pages shy of completion. Like so many other aspects of my life, it is stupidly difficult to remain consistent with anything. Reading books is no different. I've gone on streaks of knocking out 60 pages a day to barely picking it up a week at a time. Sounds like working out, but I'll get to that part later probably. It's not that it's a bad book, I like it more than *The Outsider*, but it's a typical King novel. It's certainly not a laborious read, but at times the amount of supernatural stuff does get a little much, no matter how much I need to suspend my sense of reality. One day I'll finish it and will then get to decide what to read next.

I'm not without possibilities on what to read next. The entire back of my desk is lined with books. Some of which I'll be mailing back soon, such as my Japanese books. There has come a decision, and I'm afraid it is not the easy kind, that I simply will not be getting to do everything I want while here. Of course one of these things was to learn Japanese. There are just not enough blocks of time in my day to dedicate to the task. Plus, I think it would be kind of fun to learn Japanese with the boys. Josiah probably knows way more than me, but there is definite hope with Atticus and Baby #3.

Getting to that, Saori and I still have not settled on a name. She thought Aslan would stick because I recommended it, but I had to renege. Honestly it is a noble name, but I have trouble simply pronouncing it. Tonight we went back and forth for about 40 minutes trying to resettle on something. Who knows, maybe we will compromise and agree on Aslan after all. The beauty and power of marriage.

One thing is certain, no matter how hard I press and bring it up, there will be no son of ours named Tatanka. Although I did offer to try for baby #4 in exchange. We will probably compromise and stick with Aslan and try for baby #4 after all. The beauty and power of marriage.

My writing of *The Thirsty Camel* has continued. It is remaining popular; although self-admittedly it is getting harder to write. Some days I just have nothing. Maybe that is better though because it lets the best ideas marinate a little longer. One thing I did do, however, was open the door on other writers to submit works of their own. So far only one person has submitted, LT Scott Byrd, and it was pretty funny.

The pen that just died and the one I'm writing with now are from the same pack, given to me by LCDR Tom Warner. So yes, I am thankful for the little things and fully expect this bad boy to carry the weight of my entries until I return to Japan.

I am finding myself doing my own laundry more often. There really is an odor to our free service laundry the hospital provides. I don't know; if I wake up early enough it gives me something to do while I read my book. I have to get up at 0400 though to make it worth my time. Anything later and it becomes too hot for me to sit there and read. Never would I ever dream of considering leaving my laundry unattended. Right when you're not looking is when clothes grow legs and go for a pack of smokes never to return.

I am falling deeper into the rabbit hole of smoking addiction. Because I know I can quit, even if it is mildly uncomfortable, I know I will be okay when I return. The hardest thing about it though is the shaming I get from non-smokers, and it really is not a cheap habit.

One thing I am not happy about is the mail service. I sent a letter to Baraboo almost a month ago. I understand snail mail takes longer, but really? Plus, Mail Call is only one day a week now. Besides Amazon, my most frequent mail correspondent has actually been my Grandma and Grandpa Pape in Sauk City, WI. To be honest, I am mildly surprised about how little mail I have gotten from everyone. Maybe they're just used to me being gone anyway? They definitely have no clue how much I appreciate the written letter, no matter how much of a stress reliever it is to me by writing them, there is a joy beyond words in getting them.

I did however get a letter from my dad in the form of a text message. He was replying that he had gotten my letter, and in order for history to remember his words I shall reprint them here. One thing to remember, he isn't a man of many words, and I think when God created him, he missed the sentimental gene completely. That's why it was so meaningful to read the following:

Hi Calvin. Hope you are doing well. Just got home and read your letter that arrived today. Kinda made me want to cry too. In a way it made me sad, but in a way happy to know that you're becoming a softy as you get older. Glad to see it's not taking as long as it took me. You do keep making me proud even though I don't tell you enough. I love you too son. Dad.

If history never finds what I wrote to him, I would be okay with that. Those words are for him only and anyone can infer what I probably said, though my mother on the other hand is quite the chatty Cathy when she has the time to spare. She sent a ginormous email, which I didn't mind, and she said a lot of insightful things.

Maybe the most noteworthy response to her many topics was about her not seeing herself living in Baraboo in about 10 years. I mentioned that I would be sad to not have a "home" anymore but yielded to the realization that it was a home for a family to be raised in and not for aging empty-nesters. What I wrote next even surprised myself. Before she even asked, I told her I would not want to buy the house from them when the time came for them to move along.

For the record, this is my final page in the 11-page marathon. So I've realized my goals to align with the time I still have here. Although I alluded to it earlier with the Japanese, I am getting more focused on the most bang for my buck while here. Of course I will continue to journal, but I do not intend to transcribe my work here. Putting everything on Google Docs will need to wait for post-production after I return.

Again, we've been over the Japanese bit in the previous pages, but I think I keep bringing it up because I was really looking forward to it.

Another thing I won't change or alter is reading. If anything, I need to do more of it. Working on my recognition packages, professional writing, correspondence, and learning as much as I can from Ying and Yang.

The latest word is there are going to be some big changes in Kandahar soon. How they will affect Role III is anyone's guess, but it can be a safe assumption that if there is an X-Ray Rotation, we'll need an asterisk to describe it.

My hand is very much cramped, but I'm happy to be back on the original trajectory. On July 3 to 4 we went into River City. Our first American KIA. UTV roll-over. Sad.

Postscript: At first I remembered feeling very inconvenienced that the base shut down the Wi-Fi and no email traffic was permitted. July 4, after all, is my son's birthday. Then I woke up and realized that an American was killed. Another parent back home is getting a different kind of phone call. No matter how bad you have it, someone has it worse. I eventually was able to call, and I remember it being a sobering conversation. I felt angry that Saori was telling me these first world problems and a mother's son wasn't coming home. Saori didn't know, and I didn't have much to tell her. Even if I did, OPSEC, or Operational Security, would have prevented me from disclosing much. Even if I did have more facts, to what gain would it have been to share? No entry ran longer than this one. Who knows what got into me? I think when I look back on it, the "perfect" writing condition is needed. The lighting needs to be right; the desk must be comfortable. The timing needs to be appropriate. This was a continuous uphill battle.

8 July 2020
Day 142

Here we are back on track to one page in a sitting. Only a matter of time before I disappoint myself, but for today I am happy.

I actually really liked today because I was able to knock out a couple of errands that have been put off for too long. First, I went to the post office. In a weird way, I always enjoy going to the post office. I'd compare it to my joy with going to the library, and that is probably because it reminds me of my Grandma Mongin. Anyway, I mailed two boxes back to Japan of stuff I shipped here that I now realize I never should have mailed out here to begin with.

Next, I got my haircut. Is it called a haircut when it's buzzed completely off? My favorite part is when the barber is done, and he sprays a cloth with rubbing alcohol then rubs my head.

After that I went to "wing day" at the galley. Was not totally onboard with it and did not anticipate waiting in line again for chicken wings. Then I read my book, took a nap, called the boys, slept some more, and by

2030 I was at the hospital working on stuff to improve my Sailor of the Month prospects.

Wanted to mail my college transcripts to the Navy, but it cost $12.50 per copy plus a $2.50 electronic handling fee. Tomorrow is a perfect day for that. Now I'm doing laundry in the still of the night.

Postscript: There were some guys who were all about Wing Day at the DFAC. It may have been why they continued to wake up each morning, to get back to Wednesday. I like wings, but not enough to build my reputation around. To think of it, designated days at the DFAC were probably more important than I give it credit. We all know Taco Tuesday. We just discussed Wing Wednesday. Friday was steak and crab legs. When we didn't have much going for us, it was the little things that mattered the most.

9 July 2020
Day 143

I didn't get much sleep last night, but as of now I am not feeling drained. Must be the motivation and realized focus. When I got home after doing my laundry I read until about 0215. After tossing and turning for probably 45 minutes, I woke up at 0735 to catch the bus ten minutes later for work.

Although I will probably jinx myself, there are no admitted patients, so I worked on a non-resident training course for most of the day: Safety Supervisor. There is currently a goldmine of potential with what to do.

That was all said to say this, Master Chief Branch wrote back. In true form, he asked to speak over the phone. Hopefully in less than 12 hours I will have a good conversation. I've been calling him the Geppetto of my career because as of right now, he is the puppet master. A term I'm sure he would rather not prefer, but how it should be inferred is that I have a lot of trust in him and willingly remain suspended until I get further guidance.

A lot of supply came in the back half of the afternoon. LCDR Deguzman didn't leave until close to 2000, which was late even for him. The evening has flown by and I'm looking forward to bed. Tomorrow will be a big day if only because I do not ever find myself bored.

Oh! I sent my college transcripts to the Navy today so there's that.

Postscript: Who wouldn't like to work at a hospital without any patients? I do not know if the other rotations ever had this sort of breather, but we certainly had them at Whiskey Rotation. The idle time left for many personalities to emerge and consequently contrast with others. We were not worked to the bone and fought off our own exhaustion. I'm writing about sending my college transcripts to the Navy and reading until two in the morning.

10 July 2020
Day 144

It feels like a lot has happened today, but it will probably take only a page to explain it all. Master Chief Branch and I talked on the phone. A few things to take away from the conversation. First, they were using last cycle's MAP package, but only edited that I was on deployment. What needs to happen fast is I need to assemble not only the best bragsheet of what I did here but will need to review my last Sasebo bragsheet. Everything will need to be submitted to HMCM Branch.

It feels though that they actually have nothing and I'm starting over from scratch if they submit anything at all for me. Of course, I'll never prove it, so I will have to keep faith.

Today I had my career development board, or CDB. Mine felt long at 50 minutes. It would not be a CDB if they could not find a few things to remind me where I need correction. We talked about my physical fitness, of course, but deservingly so. HM1 Wilson was present, and he said he couldn't ask me to be a better worker and had no recommendations.

One deviation I expect to do is write my goals for the day in my journal in the morning. This should help hold myself accountable instead of writing my day's failures. I played basketball with five other guys, and I felt it. What I also felt was my shorts rip right down the crotch. Just great, but I shall adapt and overcome. #mynavyexchange.com

Postscript: There are a number of episodes in the television show Dragon Ball Z *where the hero, Goku, goes into a time capsule. He can train for a year in this capsule, and when he leaves it only a day has passed in the real world. Every day I hoped my deployment would have been like that. There was a lot of buildup of potential. The trick was turning that potential into kinetic energy. Sometimes it worked, and other times I looked back and wondered what I did with my time. I take Career Development Boards very seriously because I don't believe I know everything. Someone might have a kernel of insight that I could take that would be the missing component to a much larger story. I was appreciative that the men of many rates, PS2 Bobby Krombach, HM1 David Woolen, and HM1 Jake Wilson, took the time to help me out.*

11 July 2020
Day 145

If today had to be judged, I would think that this could actually be considered a bad one. Not part of the grade, I decided to use a leftover journal for my daily goals. After one day I was able to complete all three of my goals. Couple things with that, I probably won't dwell on the "goal journal" too much in this journal, but I did establish that it does exist. Secondly, as I get more comfortable with it, I hope to expand my number of goals for each day.

I thought this day would be used for reading. I'm in the final 100 pages of *Dr. Sleep*, but I read perhaps 10 before I took a nap. Is a four-hour nap just my body telling me something else?

Was almost late to the CO call that told us nothing, but still, who wants to be "that guy"? Apparently, me. Then I left my Common Access Card at home so I could not log into a computer to work on anything else. In other words, I wasted a day to work.

Basketball went alright, but my conditioning was shit I've come to realize. That should surprise no one, but what was encouraging was I felt some obvious potential. Just have to be consistent.

I wrote a card for the family back in Japan and sent my cousin Emilia Pape a letter. I don't even know if she knows what a letter is, let alone cursive.

Postscript: I really enjoyed playing basketball. It was a great exercise, but more importantly there was a social aspect that I had been missing. Each evening we would play, and I got to hang out with a clique that I previously wasn't a part of. It was what was needed, but as we will see COVID took even that away from me.

THE PHARMACIST

Everyone has a boss. In my case, the boss was the pharmacist. Because I worked primarily at small clinics, I worked with one pharmacist at a time. All were memorable in some way. They all knew pharmacy, but it's the jelly between the bread that makes the difference.

My first pharmacist was Lieutenant Linh Quach. He rode me more than any of the pharmacists I have ever worked for. Looking back on it, my performance rated such attention. In my two years in Sasebo, I spent two months working outside of the clinic: a month in Diego Garcia and another month at Naval Hospital Yokosuka. There are only two reasons why someone is sent TAD (Temporary Assigned Duty): to showcase your best pony in front of other commands or to get the dirtbag out of your hair. Guess which one I always have assumed I was?

Lieutenant Quach was promoted to Lieutenant Commander while in Sasebo. He was from Vietnam and would always tell me that they can take your rank, your pay, and even your job, but they can't take away your education. At the time I did not like my boss. He was always telling me to practice my calculation and always left a single hair on his chin. I was looking for ways to make fun of him because I didn't understand the guy let alone myself. One day he wanted to show me a picture of his childhood home. It was a three room "house" made with cinder blocks, dirt floors and no roof. Then it hit me. He had come from next to nothing, worked his way to earn a commission, and was now an O-4 in the United States Navy.

There are no pharmacists on the US Navy ships (unless you include the two hospital ships, but they are white, and not haze gray & underway). I was the only pharmacy representative on an aircraft carrier. All the officers had cute little monikers for their titles. The AirBoss was in charge of the flight line. The GunBoss was in charge of the ammunition. Cheng was the Chief Engineer. I took it upon myself to give my own call sign: PharmBoss. Although it didn't catch on with the leadership, it was popular in the enlisted ranks, especially during ship-wide drills when I was tasked to train the stretcher bearers and main medical gear locker personnel.

Naval Branch Clinic Iwakuni had two pharmacists during my time there: Lieutenant Rachel Lantieri and Lieutenant Commander Brian Ihlenfeld. Rachel is now separated, and Brian is retired. Both were helpful in helping me chart my course. Rachel was diligent, charismatic, and let me operate with a much longer leash. The ship helped set me straight on how to be a good worker and pharmacy tech. Rachel was as close to being a friend as an officer and enlisted can get. In a sense, we were all that we had because there was only one tech and one pharmacist.

Brian was stoic and reserved. He wouldn't say much, but I know that if I ever become President of the United States, I will appoint him as my Secretary of the Interior. When asked what his qualifications were, he said that he was an Eagle Scout. He calls the position a dream job because he would get to tour the National Parks and hang out with Smokey the Bear at press briefs. If he only knew that Smokey was under the Secretary of Agriculture.

Back in Sasebo, I had three pharmacists. As of this writing, they are all still active duty. Some were passive, none were aggressive. Some led, some existed. To be a pharmacist in Sasebo meant to be the quasi-psychologist because they had their own office with enough room in it for one desk and chair. I certainly logged enough time to let them know where my mind was at throughout certain points.

We had one pharmacist in Afghanistan, Commander Vince Deguzman. To say he was the best pharmacist I ever worked for would not be fair to those I spent more time with, but he certainly left an impression that will not be soon forgotten. If I put a label on a vial crooked, he would tell me that it did not look pharmaceutically elegant. If I was over my head with inpatient calculations, he'd come in in the middle of the night after putting in a full day. In my end of deployment gift to myself, the book, he addressed me as "HM1" and that was not by mistake. He was the kind of leader that would tell you what you needed to know, but what was done in rooms I wasn't part of was where he did most of his work.

What struck me most about CDR Deguzman was his work ethic. He was at work every day. The technicians rotated days. He was working on things back at his parent command, present command at the hospital, and setting up his future as he was coming into his orders window simultaneously. He was the reason I qualified for my Lean Six Sigma greenbelt certificate, putting in more time than was expected, let alone necessary.

One thing I will always take away with me was the day he was promoted to O-5, or Commander. He became a senior officer that day. It is a hard accomplishment to achieve, especially for a pharmacist in the Navy. No one would have thought badly of him if he relaxed a little bit. Except he didn't. He was promoted, said some words, and went right back into the pharmacy to begin working again. When we were awarded our End of Tour (EOT) awards, he was given a high award from the Army. He didn't even say anything, and when I came into the pharmacy after eating my cake and jaw jacking with the rest of the staff, I found him working.

Then again, I shouldn't be too surprised. The man had more letters after his name than the alphabet. He has a PharmD, PhD, MBA, and a couple other academic accomplishments, some of which I had never heard of until I met him. You wouldn't know it by talking to him that he was probably the most academically accomplished man you'd ever talk to in your life. He was modest, prior enlisted, and one to be remembered for a long time.

Like the rest of the pharmacy staff, I put my foot in my mouth more times than I should have, forgetting I was talking to a senior officer, things like that. HM1 Wilson on more than one occasion had to reel me back in and put me in check. That was necessary, it was part of his job description, but it also made me feel even more terrible that it had to be directed at me. In my mind, I knew I was better than that, but keeping the tiger in the cage was and still is a constant struggle for me. I'm just thankful that there were so many who offered allowances to still see me succeed. CDR Deguzman was one of those men.

12 July 2020
Day 146

I guess today was a good day, although it was full of distractions, which I will no doubt talk about in a moment.

Pretty cool that I rode my "new" bike into work this morning. LCDR Deguzman picked up a new bike and donated his old one to me. Really, it's a functional piece of crap with crooked handlebars and one set of brakes only, but I got to work much faster. Surprised myself on my "bike muscles" being so worked. Oh well.

What I really should be doing is working on my bragsheet/MAP, but I was stunted by two things primarily: *Thirsty Camel* and a new Green Belt project. I will say now I am not thrilled with the Green Belt process. There was a lot to learn, but more specifically understanding what was missed out on. One of my goals was working to completion so I need to suck it the hell up. Such a rare opportunity that there is not only a black belt on the deployment, but he's the pharmacist.

I bought a new 5lb bag of coffee from Enderley Coffee Company. Changed up the flavor to test out what I like. May buy from them when I get back to Japan.

I was sore today and grumpier than anyone around me deserved. Being on a calorie restricted diet does not help. I think we may have decided on a first name for incoming Baby #3. After the greatest leader of the 20th century, Winston.

Postscript: This is a funny post because it reveals so much of what the future holds. In hindsight, as we shall read on, there were a lot of relevant mentions here. For example, I only buy my coffee from Enderley Coffee Co. these days. They provide excellent service, and I was thankful they could mail out to Afghanistan at all. The Green Belt saga is one that would continue until I left Kandahar. What is a Green Belt? To put it in a way I was able to understand, it's a methodology of learning the science of process improvement. It's a qualification under the Lean Six Sigma program. Yes, my third son was ALMOST named Winston, but this was the second time we felt we had a lock.

17 July 2020
Day 147, 148, 149, 150 & 151

Here I go again, letting the days slip away from me. I can't say I'm totally surprised by my behavior. Each day when it came to writing in my journal, I was so mentally fried that journaling became the last thing I wanted to do. Within the next few pages, I'll have the distinct opportunity to try and explain what it was I meant, and where I'm headed.

First though, as I write this, I'm actually sitting outside at 1300 on July 17. I admittedly have surprised myself being outside for this long with the only purpose to write. To be fair, I'm sitting in the shade on a picnic table between the two buildings of the barracks. My original intent was to peruse Google to look up literary agents, but I'll get into that more in a bit. For reasons that are left unexplained, my Chromebook was being difficult, and I had to close it for the time being. Luckily the idealist within me decided to bring other writing materials along in case I felt extra ambitious.

This morning I felt semi-motivated on my day off, even though I woke up at 1030. Showered, cleaned my room a bit (was mostly brainstorming things to mail home early really) and told myself I was going to write.

Hmm, the thought just popped into my mind, why I care so much about writing. When I could be doing a million other things from learning new skills to mindless entertainment, I hang my shingle on writing. I always enjoyed doing it but was never explicitly great at it. If my writing ever becomes renowned, one of two things will happen. First, a major case of "imposter syndrome" will fill me. The second will inspire me to advocate that if you keep looking, then someone will find you.

That's where I suppose I'm at though, but I'm balancing between professional writing and working toward getting my personal stuff recognized. The professional part is easy though, my timeline to submit my MAP package was moved up considerably. The email from Master Chief Branch came on I believe Monday or Tuesday of this week saying that instead of the end of the month, he'll need it by the end of the week.

Luckily the patient load was low, but anxiety was real high, real fast. It didn't matter if I was on shift or not, I was at the office. Trying to get this or that done.

Possibly the real excitement came because I was finally given a shot to make my argument. For the first time I had a morsel of influence on my own destiny. For that, to me, the pressure was on to prove myself.

Couple of things to unpack here. First, it was not done alone. There was of course Master Chief Branch. Then here in Afghanistan was Senior Chief Cameron Wink and even closer was HM1 Jacob Wilson. These three people would be who I'd have to blame for any "meritorious" success. The flipside of this story is I know I was never supposed to be part of this conversation to begin with. My counter to that, or at least my defense, is that ever since I came to Sasebo, at least when talking to HM2 Yani Lopez, leadership has gone out of their way to specifically ask her, but never me. Even though I had to ask, my inquiry was returned with guidance, and I could not have asked for anything more.

Of course, this could all be a big ruse from Master Chief and my email was deleted without reading it. I have to prepare myself that is a possibility. In my heart, I don't think that is both true and will happen, but at the end of the day I did my best, gave my best work. Yes, I was busy pounding out professional writing, and it may show some dividends, but like all investments, it may not bear any fruit at all.

Then there is the other side of the house. My personal time. *Doctor Sleep* is now finished. Typical Stephen King. The movie, much different story. My brother Dylan said not to hold my breath, and he was right. The first two acts of the film were adopted from the book, and the director did what he could. The third act followed the 1980 movie of *The Shining*. This makes sense, but I think it could have used a R-rating. Come to think of it, all horror movies should have a R-rating.

Then I started reading a book Dylan got me for Christmas a few years ago, *The Best of the Harvard Lampoon*. I did not like it. At first, I thought it was because I didn't understand humor back at the turn of the 20th century. So, I flipped forward to modern writing and still did not find it funny. Will thank my brother and will move on.

Now I'm reading *Going to Wisconsin Gold: Stories of our State Olympians.* So far, I am finding it interesting. It is a collection of mini biographies, so it was a nice little book. Of course, I'll say it shouldn't take long, but will probably take much longer than necessary.

Then there is the fun side of my personal time. I started to cold call some literary publishing agents about their interest in representing a memoir of an Afghan Combat Hospital. Despite my minimal effort, I received one reply. It was a polite "get bent" response, but one I will save for the day I do make it.

In an interesting turn of events, I have been emailing my godmother and only other published author of the family, Aunt Laura Erickson. She has asked me the inevitable "send me what you have, and I'll take a look at it." In some ways I just become a lot more nervous. Then again, like the advice I got from a male porn star when asked, how do you know you have what it takes: if you can beat off naked in the family living room in front of everyone, then you have a shot. In other words, if I can muster the courage to show what I have and take some direction from family, then total strangers should be easy. As of now it is a fun little side project and I know if I want to get serious about it that much more work would ensue.

Oh! I spent a good amount of time on the phone with Dr. Christina "Dearest" Solomon. Many times, our talks tend to carry a theme of sorts, and our last talk was no different. She's so interesting to me and I'm always entertained when we talk. Not like seeing my boys though.

Definitely Not a Role 3 MMU Publication

The Thirsty Camel

ARE SECOND CLASSES FIGURING IT OUT?

In a shocking turn of events, it would appear the Second Classes of the Whiskey Rotation are starting to figure it out and seemingly "get along."

What started as a simple text message turned into the realization that a group of individuals coming together, aligning their goals and seeking a common vision can drastically shift a paradigm to however they choose.

"I guess we are pretty much Chiefs now," said one PO2, "we all think we work two paygrades ahead of where we are now, so it's not too far of a stretch."

With the exception of one Petty Officer with higher aspirations than the joys of working amongst peers, the rest have bit the pillow to put with one another's memes, bad jokes and "idea fairy" initiatives in the effort to promote a better rank, command and Navy.

"Everyone is free to come and go from our communal electronic gatherings, but we know that the hardest part is leading among your peers."

It has been stated in the Thirsty Camel before how competitive it can be in the "Second to None" paygrade, but when egos are set aside, it has been noted how good it actually feels to get along.

The next question is where does it go from here? How many recognition boards can we run from top to bottom? How many awards or letters can we write? What is the landscape of nurturing Sailors going to look like?

All of these questions lead to a very exciting, promising outlook for the Second Classes.

"Peer involvement should not be an issue since we are figuring it out on how if you want to go fast, go alone, but if you want to go far, go together."

AND THEY SHALL FROM TIME TO TIME, SPEAK

This is a very special issue of The Thirsty Camel. If anyone recalls the last issue, a gauntlet was cast into the lovely mess that is Whiskey Rotation to submit their own articles for publication.

Some of you deemed yourselves worthy of this task, and picked Mjölnir up. We are proud to announce at the Thirsty Camel some articles were from the People of Whiskey besides the usual suspects of The Camel staff.

And they shall from time to time submit original work from the deckplates. It has been reviewed, revised when needed and reprinted for the masses to see.

We at the Thirsty Camel are proud to have grown so much that a following has started, and we wish to reward this patronage to the fullest extent. Here and henceforth, expect to see different styles of humor, perspectives and context.

In order to protect those with the best of intentions, articles will remain anonymous and continue to fall under the Thirsty Camel umbrella. This should promote a fearless populous to offer their best work without reprisal, retribution and all those other good terms CMEO loves to worry about.

Do not go quietly into the night, and enjoy. The invitation remains open for all.

Vol I Issue VII

No one knows when this was published and we assure you that no one cares either.

Special points of interest:

- What matters most is how well you walk through the fire.
- No one cares, work harder.
- If you're so smart, why aren't you winning?
- Courage is what it takes to stand up and speak, but also to sit down and listen.

Inside this issue:

Southern Nectar	2
Crisis in Pharmily	2
Inside Story	2
Injury on the Court	3
Inside Story	3
COT's Delusion	3
Camel's Moby Dick	4
Hairy Bacon	4
Mr. Chow Hates COVID	4

IF IT CAN HAPPEN TO WILFORD BREMELY, IT CAN GET YOU TOO, MAKE NO MISTAKE.

OUTBREAK OF TYPE II DIABETES: LT BYRD TEA LINKED

As Role 3 is fighting its own war against the imaginary COVID-19, the PAD and other ancillary services are struggling with a war their own.

It was first noticed a few weeks ago when it became clear the PAD crew was taking way too many bathroom breaks. At first attributed to over-hydration, it quickly became apparent that something much more serious was at hand.

HM3 Alden, the most unhealthy Corpsman within the Whiskey rotation realized something was wrong when his vision started getting more and more blurry. Simply attributing it to lack of sleep, he did what any red-blooded American would. He slammed another glass of Southern nectar and got back to work.

HM3 Gibford, who recently reported tingling in his feet, thought it was related to sitting for hours on end doing absolutely nothing. A quick Google search led him to WebMD, the most trusted source of medical knowledge here in southern Afghanistan. Dry mouth, weight loss, fatigue, headaches - were these related to KAF or something else?

HM2 Slagle, aka Ari Gold, mandated finger sticks for his entire crew in an attempt to get ahead of this epidemic. While we can't report the exact results due to HIPPA, a source did say the sugars ranged from 145-360. We at Role 3 ain't got time for that. Hopefully General Eastman doesn't find out.

If you want to give the sweet, delicious brown liquid a try, a fresh batch is rumored to be made every Tuesday. LT Byrd's sweet southern sun tea makes Red Diamond taste like gutter water and Gold Peak has already offered to buy the recipe.

LT Byrd could not be reached for comment. He's got S*&T to do. The Camel was able to talk to LT Hollins, the most important unimportant person at Role 3, and he stated he has repeatedly asked LT Byrd to change the recipe. If not for him, then for the kids.

NEAR MISS: CRISIS IN THE PHARMACY

Thirsty Camel beat writers state the phamily considered calling in a mostly worthless "Red Dot" WhatsApp message to assist in their endeavor

ICU nurses are collecting donations to purchase a calculator and pill-splitter for the powder monkeys in the Pharmacy.

Despite claiming the strength of optimus maximus and intellect of Sir Isaac Newton, the phamily staff were unable to solve the Gordian Knot of transforming a 15mg tablet of the NSAID meloxicam into a 7.5mg tablet.

Reports obtained by the Thirsty Camel beat writers state the phamily considered calling in a mostly worthless "Red Dot" WhatsApp message to assist in their endeavor, but were stood down by the ICU oberführer Winfield Scott Byrd.

LT Byrd, already on the Executive Officer's shitlist for giving half of PAD TOC Type II diabetes, smartly consulted with supervisor, LCDR Valencia "Dream" Weaver, who defused the potentially explosive situation by cutting the aforementioned tablet in half with a knife found in the Role 3 galley.

Bravo Zulu to LCDR Weaver to have the fortitude for such a courageous act!

DCSS was not available for comment because he was rolling with his blowup "jiu jitsu" doll. HM1 Wilson could not be bothered while playing basketball, and HM1 LaPenna said something in literal Greek at his "off-site" office.

Only HM2 Rastall was seen in the pharmacy which should not surprise anyone. He offered a tip of the hat to the ICU staff too.

LaPENNA AND ▇▇▇▇ ON KAF'S MOST WANTED LIST

Don't be a Muma, and definitely do not be a LaPenna.

HN Dreadin and Valdez can exhale a sign of relief now that Whiskey's two newest boots have been identified.

On just another, routine day of duty, two Sailors had to learn the hard lesson of not running through the motions of being a watchstander. Although the details will remain sealed under the entitlement of rank and position in the organizational chart, what can be heavily suggested is there may have been a high speed chase involving the Provost Marshal Officer, who is already quite familiar with Role 3 due to LCDR Salazar's spunky defiance of authority.

Executive Officer CAPT Jeff Klinger could not be more proud.

With a wad of sweet leafy tobacco, the XO may have stated that he could not any more proud of the team.

"I really don't know what I do every day anyway, so when these problems arise, I feel useful. Role 3 needs more rebels."

Wear your masks and if you're going to drive, bring your license. "It won't happen to me" is a dumb excuse.

HM2 MUTOMBO HAS X-RAY ON HAND

The Sailor previously known as Robinson has morphed into HM2 Mutombo.

Reports conclude that HM2 was taken into the radiology suite late last evening to obtain imaging of his possibly broken hand.

Mutombo was thought to injure the hand during a pickup basketball game when he swatted one of HM1 Kubil layups into the next time zone.

Although a rare occurrence to see the laboratory LPO utterly humiliated, there is precedence. The Thirsty Camel previously reported on Kubil losing in a game of horse to HM1 Jacob Wilson.

Good people bounce back. Sometimes because they are jiggly and buoyant. Other times because they are so chiseled they push the rest of the world down upon impact. This is the case for the DMS LPO.

A man of many titles, Petty Officer Kubil reportedly sent flowers and fruit basket to the injured basketball assassin.

HM2 Mutombo, a scholar and gentleman, did not know that to think, but his mind was already back to figuring out how to help out the Sailors at Whiskey Rotation by standing up the highly anticipated Enlisted Advancement Program. Also known as EAP, HM2 has put in a considerable amount of time in developing a strategy to best aid not only his subordinate Sailors, but peers as well.

The initiative is being received with open arms, too. One Goat Locker inductee said, "We appreciate when HM2 is not injuring himself while embarrassing clinic staff, and focuses his attention on adding value to the mission."

Hands will heal. Pride will recover, but teamwork will live on.

Should have obtained rights for this one.

HM2 ROBINSON GIVING HM1 KUBIL THE FAMOUS FINGER WAVE

MAIL CALL DAY SANCTION AS KAF HOLIDAY

Each and every Monday, provided the plane lands the day prior, the crew at Role 3 gets more excited than normal.

Said one brainy director, "Mass Casualties don't even get the crew this fired up."

Typically Monday is not a very positive day of the week. Back stateside having a "case of the Mondays" is more contagious than COVID. Back home, morale reaches an all-time low on Monday.

Well, we aren't in America, and this isn't a typical life. Monday has been rechristened as a quasi-holiday from this moment forward.

Although the authority to declare these types of observances remains hazy, HM3 Vo said that he will shoulder the burden of proclaiming Mail Call Day a revolving holiday.

Unfortunately a Camel's favorite day of the week is already on the public register, but should Hump Day ever be switched, he would choose Monday because of Mail Call.

"Morale just rockets on Monday, and it really speaks to how ass-backwards this place actually is," expanded the brainy director.

Let us all pray the Dear John letters stay at home, and the candy comes in full. We shall rejoice in the many care packages that come our way, and may the black liquor ice stay away.

And don't forget to tip your mail orderlies. That collateral blows.

"Morale just rockets on Monday, and it really speaks to how ass-backwards this place actually is"

COT CONFIRMS RESEMBELENCE TO BECKHAM

The Camel's investigation division has reported that at the COT's insistence, he recently received a 2nd confirmation of his close resemblance to British hero and MLS gold-digger David Beckham.

Long suspected, but now obvious narcissistic tendencies of our fearless COT may be clouding his otherwise clear memory, but he states that upon receiving his 1st haircut here in Afghanistan, his extra thirsty barber exclaimed, "You look just like David Beckham!"

COT also reports an eerily identical incident at his home barbershop in Eagle, Idaho (not to be confused with Yudaho, IA) going back about 5 years ago.

His wife at the time, the ever-honest lass she was reportedly cried, "Fertilizer! [sic]," but the Chief of Trauma was not deterred.

After all, COT was clear to pull no punches that his wives, all three of them, were never capable of appreciating his chiseled and sporting demeanor the way he deserved.

It should be made as clear as can be that there are in fact slight differences between Beckham and himself. Most of which, one is known to move around for a living while the other jockeys a desk as he fights the urge to insert copious amounts of Preparation H at inopportune times, like BOD meetings.

And one is married to Posh Spice, so there's that too.

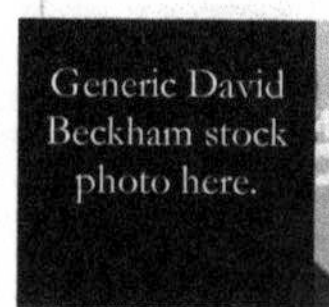
Generic David Beckham stock photo here.

"Commander Mayberry"

███ HAIRY SECRET COMES TO LIGHT IN WAKE OF FACTS

Whiskey softy and all around good guy HM3 ███ in PAD TOC has always been good at keeping secrets. It's one of the beautiful things about him and his friendship with others.

It should not come to anyone's surprise then that the story behind that borderline unauthorized haircut of his shares another deep and dark secret.

Rumor has it that Petty Officer ███ is able to keep that mane looking sleek and slick is by stealing the bacon grease from the Role 3 galley on some mornings.

To prove this conjecture, HM3 was heard to offer anyone smell his hair to prove that it has the odor of bacon. To wit, keep tabs on the level of shagginess and lack of upkeep the farther out from "bacon" day we get.

The use of bacon grease was suppose to counter the smell of dried sea water from his days at BUD/S, and the habit stuck ever since.

MR. CHOW IS NOT IMPRESSED WITH COVID

Did you know that the actor who plays Mr. Chow in the Hang Over movies is an actual doctor. It's true, look it up. Anyway, can't afford the rights to the photo for a cheap laugh here.

Our laboratory's finest, Mr. Chow is done with COVID testing.

This became clear when the Las Vegas mafia wannabe and part-time day trader was seen on the smoke deck and literally nowhere else.

"When I grow up, like at all, you know, like my height and not my maturity, I want to chase the markets and get involved with syndicated crime out in a desert," said Mr. Chow.

He is in luck with the being in the desert part of his fantasy. As long as we don't go into River City, he can continue chasing the markets, too. Go Mr. Chow, Go!

Being Sailor of the Whatever is a high honor and Mr. Chow is not taking the burden lightly.

He celebrates by burning the cheapest cigarettes the Pilipino market can offer, but if sharing means caring then he is the best guy on the deployment to have as a friend.

At the end of the day, Mr. Chow hates COVID because it means it has to detract from what he wants to do, but he does it because damn it feels good to be American!

REEDER IS NOW THE CAMEL'S MOBY DICK

Some stock photo of Moby Dick going to town on a little fishing boat. Was a cool photo though.

THE ELUSIVE WHALE WILL ONE DAY BE THE TROPHY THE CAMEL ALWAYS WANTED

LT Sam Reeder is the white whale which haunts the Camel. After seven issues, and hours of observing the crew at Whiskey one thing has become apparent, some are the low hanging fruit, and others are harder than Chinese algebra to catch.

Not without trying, The Camel has yet to catch Dr. Reeder in the act of doing anything newsworthy. There was that one movie night, but really not one thing to peg her with or make fun of her for.

Although there is much speculation as to why this is, some guesses include that as an Emergency Department physician, she is out exercising during working hours.

Another suggestion is she is in the back room hatching an evil plan on how to torment the nurses of the ICU. Like a rapper, with a pen and pad working on anything besides work. As if she is trying to launch a satirical newsletter of her own.

A third option is a perfectly timed evacuation plan from the Camel's line of sight. Like, she can hear the ground trembling, and she knows to dip out, like a spec ops roll-out maneuver in the movies.

All of these theories are not above serious consideration, but the reality is Dr. Reeder is probably doing a solid job training her Corpsman, inviting other members of the crew to learn and getting everyone as cross-trained as possible in the anticipation of the next colossal event.

Maybe she is out slaying as the Fun Boss, writing to companies and advocating for our morale. These are just thoughts, however.

Do not be confused, if she ever leaves a gun outside or something she's going to make PAO's Normandy look like paintball.

Harpooning one of Whiskey's biggest performers that isn't named Wilson would be the story of the deployment. These are the facts, and the Camel never fabricates truth.

Until then, we can all be thankful that she's out here killing it, enriching our lives if even at the margin, or one cross-fit WOD at a time, whichever will have you.

WHISKEY HELPS.

18 July 2020
Day 152

Today is my duty day, and I thought I was a productive member of society. For one, and maybe the dark horse of the things to brag about, is I'm enjoying my new Audible title. It's a Great Lecture Series called *The Deceptive Mind: A Scientific Guide to Critical Thinking Skills*. I started listening to it after HM1 LaPenna left for the day, but HM1 Wilson came in a bit later, so I told him what I was listening to. He said I have the things in place to do some really great things, and that felt good.

Today I climbed back on the treadmill. Maybe it was the new playlist of music, or maybe I can blame the five days or so of rest, but I slayed. Time was 60:00. Distance was 4.57 miles, and the calorie count was 1,125. I think the best part was my nonstop pace of 21:00, up from 17:00 at a 5.0 speed.

I also started building my official Sailor of the Month package. It's coming along nicely, but what I really need to do is bite the pillow on my Green Belt projects for Lean Six Sigma. If I can knock these out before we leave, I'll be extremely proud of myself.

We had a mass casualty drill today, and it could have gone better. I thought there were too many observers who got in the way, and the other half wasn't present, like lab, because they had actual work to do.

Looking forward to hearing back from Aunt Laura who promised to be "brutally honest."

Postscript: This was during the hottest days of the year. Besides playing basketball, I did not go outside during the day to exercise, especially in Swole 3. For other guys, the makeshift gym was their sanctuary; it was the equivalent to my writing. In the hospital, we had one treadmill, and that is what I used when I did want to sweat. Inside of the boardwalk, a shell of itself, was a quarter-mile track and artificial-turf soccer field. At night when I couldn't sleep, I would go out there, or sometimes I'd go with LT Byrd if he felt like having company, but I generally exercised by myself; mostly because I was too embarrassed to do it in front of others.

19 July 2020
Day 153

What a crappy day. I definitely either woke up on the wrong side of the bed or someone boldly pissed in my corn flakes. (Speaking of, normal Corn Flakes with that rooster sound rather appealing).

It all started at 0330 when an ER patient came for non-serious meds. You are welcome for my service, unnamed Sergeant. At the same time, we were placed on standby for a gunshot wound to the arm, possible amputation. They didn't come until 0700, so I slept for another hour.

It got a little crazy but was sorted out. All I wanted to do was complete my Sailor of the Month package, then be on my merry way after hitting the treadmill. I left at 1300 more flustered than I've been in a long time. HM1 Wilson just wouldn't drop his enthusiasm about going to lift weights with him. I hate lifting iron. I killed it on the treadmill yesterday but did not have follow-up success. Only 40:00, 3.0 miles and 800 calories. I thought jogging would help me blow off steam, but it hardly put a dent in my mood.

Ended my workday by copping off to LCDR Deguzman who was offering another way for me to do something to help myself. Ultimately, I feel like I'm failing because I'm not keeping up with the help offered and it hurts.

Postscript: As mentioned before, the gym was a ritual to some people. Those people, unlike me, probably didn't need to go to the gym, but that was because they went every day. It was a part of their social routine; a way to blow off the day's steam and build comradery. I was too self-conscious to objectively think that because they were actively wanting me to join them, it was because they were okay with watching me fail. It meant that I was growing. This is a classic example of refusing the help that was selflessly offered, and deep down inside I felt terrible about it.

20 July 2020
Day 154

Before I get too unmotivated, let me jot a few lines, which may fall under another eye one day. My day started early, ended long, but it's not even 2200 yet. Allow me to elaborate.

Biggest Loser weigh-in was today at 0900. I made it on time. The scale we used was nifty because it calculated a lot more than weight. The scale did Body Mass Index and a few more metrics. Afterwards, I used the scale I normally do, and I came in at 285 lb. That's four pounds less than my last weigh-in a week ago.

Went to the treadmill again today. I think this was my third straight day. Although I increased my non-stop time to 23:00, I was only on for 32:00 and 700 calories. My calorie-restricted diet might be catching up because I was drained.

Mail Call today, and it did not disappoint. Big Dan's care package arrived, and it included pretty much every damn thing I asked for, including the taste of Christmas, Djarome Blacks. Doctor Christina "Dearest" Solomon's epistle came too. She included two WWI contrasting poems. They were a delight to read! Headphones and moleskin and boot socks came from Amazon. Received an email from Grandma Pape too, and I replied.

Besides doing my laundry, the capstone to my day was working on my Lean Six Sigma project. The outline is done, just need to put on a computer.

Postscript: "Big Dan" Schrickel is a guy who could have an entire chapter dedicated to him. He was a chum back in my UW-Green Bay days, and we've kept in touch all these years later. I was feeling down and sorry for myself, so I gave him a call. Within 36 hours his care package was in the mail. The letters received in Afghanistan have all been kept and are now cataloged in my personal collection. It started in 4th grade, or 1997, when my family moved to Tennessee. They hold a particular place close in my heart.

21 July 2020
Day 155

Here is a bit of unexpected news, we are only five days away from earning the deployment ribbon. Here I thought it was 90 days since living in Afghanistan, but I was told that it's actually since our time in Qatar. So there's that.

Today was slow, but still frustrating. I was able to work on *The Thirsty Camel* and only have three articles left to finish. Hopefully they will be reserved for guest articles. I have a feeling I'm going to really like this one. I've given myself time to revise and edit.

We had to do an inventory on all our COVID IV fluids that have been spread out across the hospital. By we, I mean me, and it sucked. There were like 105 cases altogether that I shuffled around and took notes of.

Had to make a couple IVs in the hood for our admitted patients, and I stumbled. In a way, I would say that I've been rusty. Another argument is I wasn't focused, which can actually be dangerous, so I know I can do better. LCDR Deguzman was there. HM1 Wilson is doing a good job, to his sincere credit, pointing out when I'm not talking to officers correctly, especially our pharmacist. It's helping me realize why I'm such a turn-off to the brass back in Sasebo.

Saori and I had an interesting talk. I expressed my concerns about preparedness for the baby.

Postscript: Medical errors happen all the time. Mostly it is caused by complacency by the healthcare professional. It was touched on previously, but this is another example. The pharmacy team was a little strange because there were only three techs, and I was the lowest rank as a 12-year Second Class. It made for some humbling situations doing menial work such as tracking all those cases of IV fluids. Rank definitely has its privileges, or RHIP.

22 July 2020
Day 156

Today is a day I really do not feel like writing, but these are the times which try a man's soul. Just because I'm tired does not mean I should let myself off so easily. After last night's journal entry, I did three things. The first: told myself to get comfy with a book. I fell down the YouTube rabbit hole instead. Second, I said I was going to bed at a decent hour so I wouldn't be up all night being hungry. Instead, I dug into the snack drawer and indulged. Third, I finally talked to Rich, on the day his cat died. The only positive from that was it took attention away from me having to talk about the deployment.

After a day of rest on the treadmill, I was back, and the results were good. Like KAF's personal record. Time 60:00, distance 4.65 miles and calorie count was 1,132. Previous distance personal record was 4.57 and calorie count was 1,125 set on 18 July.

Although I didn't leave the hospital until almost 2000, 37 hours after arriving, I felt accomplished because I finished the first leg of the Lean Six Sigma project. I also knocked out another *Camel* article, leaving two to go. Will probably publish tomorrow.

Was allowed to review some correspondence for HM1 Wilson, too. It's that part of being a Petty Officer I enjoy the most and miss.

Postscript: This day highlights one task after another. I really appreciated HM1 Wilson trusting me to review some work. Maybe it was because he didn't want to do it, but it took me away from doing E-3 level work. I felt important and to me it was meaningful. There was always something to do but remaining focused was a constant battle. I went to bed tired but fulfilled.

THE THIRSTY CAMEL

Published when it was meant to, no date required, or necessary

Definitely Not a Role 3 MMU Publication

Issue # VIII

Points to Ponder:

- One-way ticket to Mast if you rough up the Role 3 Library.
- The irony of tobacco cessation campaign coming out of the pharmacy is not lost.
- Be glad you look ugly. Lots of people will never get the chance you have.
- It's scientifically impossible to have a bad interaction with HM1 Woolen...and also say "bunny" angrily.

Inside this issue:

XO's Decision	2
Actual Wilson Article	2
Half-Squat Science	2
Self and PMO	3
Jenga Champ	3
SEA Call	3
Cup of Joe Award	4
Mail Bag	4

THE CAMEL ENTERS INTO THE "BIGGEST LOSER" CONTEST

Standby for heavy rolls, rather literally this time around. The Thirsty Camel has thrown its three humps and hat into the arena by announcing that they will in fact be competing in the "Biggest Loser" competition.

This has long been expected, as the Great Humped One has been saddling up for this showdown of showdowns for some time now.

The Camel's roommate has cited the local legend has been saying their prayers and eating its vitamins at night.

Hulkamania has been renamed "Camelmania."

There is stiff competition to deal with. Although the heavy favorites are CDR Shaieb, HM1 LaPenna and HMCS Wink, the Camel knows that in his three-sizes too big heart that if he works hard and stays away from CIO's oatmeal and raisin cookies, it could be the deciding factor.

"All he's doing is going around and reciting 'Rounders' quotes," said one member of the janitorial staff. "Apparently he is a big fan of 'Kenny KGB' because he paces back and forth talking about 'slaying a monster.'

The cerebral assassin with one of his awesome WrestleMania entrances.

The Camel entering each weigh-in

Sponsored by the Fun Boss, LT Reeder, the most important unimportant Officer LT Hollins and the rest of the MWR team, "The Biggest Loser" is intended to shock the Whiskey Rotation into believing that it is now "cutting season" before returning to our families.

The Camel is looking forward to seeing all the participation and may the odds ever be their favor, but especially his.

The Game sits upon the throne. The king of kings...hail to the King

Projected 'after-image' of the King of Kings," The Thirsty Camel

HARLEM GLOBETROTTER USO TOUR STOP CANCELLED

Do you remember the day the Whistling Died? It is written with a heavy heart that the Harlem Globetrotters will not be stopping at KAF after all.

In light of the recent announcement that there will be no more team sports authorized in the southern Afghanistan theater, the legendary basketball show group found it in thir best interest to move on from the sand box and onto other things. The troops were really looking forward to the base VIP verse Globetrotter pickup basketball game, but no one is more sick to hear the news than CAPT Daniel Kahler, who was rumored to be practicing late into the night until the order was released.

"Fertilizer" was the only word the Chief of Medicine could muster. It's certainly a new day at KAF, but it's always darkest before the dawn.

Issue #VIII was originally a special edition that complained exclusively about the Covid restrictions, and all the fun secured. This is the only remaining article of that issue.

THE THIRSTY CAMEL

Page 2

Picture of a teddy bear with a gold fouled anchor in the middle. The anchor is the symbol of Navy Chiefs.

Sample of Chief's private collection, his "comfort toy."

XO LOSES OUT ON $5000 IN LIEU OF JAW-JACKING HABIT

Role 3 Executive Officer, CAPT Jeff Klinger is not having a good day.

While making his rounds, perusing the deckplates and getting an accurate assessment of staff morale, the senior officer was locked into a lively discussion that detained him from a decision which cost him a sum of money which mattered.

Allegedly the EBay auction which would sell CAPT Klinger's Beanie Baby collection expired while his staff was chatting it up in the pharmacy like a broken carnival fortune teller about absolutely nothing of consequence. Typical pharmacy.

CAPT Klinger was beside himself, firmly believing the market was fertile enough to make a substantial profit.

This story was not without its troubles though. First, XO has denied that the Beanie Babies were actually his, but his teenage daughter's. Sources say that the teenager is too young to know how EBay actually works, but too old to find the value in the little beanie, well, babies.

The investigative team on the Thirsty Camel have uncovered that Captain Klinger lost out on $5000 in his decision to hear every pharmacy E5 brag about how they should be field promoted as if XO had anything to do with that.

Filler Picture

We all know XO loves weird things, and Beanie Babies aligns perfectly with his little kinks. Please be nice to him today, he is in a fragile place, and we need our XO happy.

He will allegedly begin trading in that non-centralized cryptocurrency rather than 90's fads.

WILSON LEARNS HOW TO LEAD BY PHONE CALLS FROM HOME

"my 6 year old pretty much talks to me the same way as my most senior Second Class Petty Officers"

Every leader has their own way. More than we want to acknowledge that way is high and right as opposed to right on the money, but DCSS LPO HM1 Jacob Wilson is squarely in the latter group.

"I learn to lead my Sailors more and more each time I call home to talk to my little girls," says the First Class Petty Officer, "my 6 year old pretty much talks to me the same way as my most senior Second Class Petty Officers, so pretty much everywhere I go, I'm learning how to become a better leader.

No doubt leading a group of opinionated, know-it-all grown ass adults can be synonymous with fatherhood. In the case that the parallel's are clear as mud, just trust the Camel on this one.

"I learned how pats on the back are important, but also I have to know when to pat a little lower and a little harder," said Wilson.

Even if HM1 can be as vexing as a 6 year old in his methodology, like a small child, his heart is pure with intentions and ultimately means well, even if a drop-kick to the face from time to time would make some subordinates dance until late into the night.

COMMANDER SHAIEB'S HALF-SQUATS ADDING UP

Think of the skinniest person you know, then drop 20lbs and that is who we are talking about

CDR SHAIEB WAS WEIRDLY NOT ON TIME FOR THIS PHOTO SHOOT SO LaPENNA IN A WIG HAD TO STAND IN HIS PLACE.

Our very own orthopedic surgeon is making big gains as Whiskey begins to creep closer to the finish line of the deployment.

CDR Mark Shaieb has been heading over to Swole 3 rather unassumingly each and every morning, and it's starting to show some progress.

Donned with his N95 3M mask and a gut full of determination, CDR has been hitting in the gym, bookending each workout with what a common on-looker may call "half-squats."

The Thirsty Camel was on the scene to ask the Officer and gentleman what the story was, from the horses mouth with the peculiar exercise routine.

"You see, if I do half squats at the beginning of the workout, and half squats at the end, it's like I'm doing a full squat"

Although this is certainly some orthopedic expert voodoo science, it should not go without saying that at least he is out there, getting it in.

A heavy favorite for the Biggest Loser competition, he is at least 1,000 squats ahead of SEA.

XO BAILS CDR SELF OUT OF PMO JAIL—NO VEHICLE OR MASK TO BE FOUND

PMO was dispatched after an elderly gentleman was spotted by the eye in the sky, KAF's own zeppelin, known as "Big Brother" for purposelessly wandering the base.

The report states that the monitors became uneasy after noticing the same person walking "all over" Kandahar Airfield.

It's become known that a figure resembling CDR Philip Self was seen near Cambridge DFAC, then an hour later he was seen walking around what used to be the Poo Pond.

Later in the night, he was spotted near ECP 5 and then over near the burn pits. At that point, fearing the subject was confused, demented, or both, "Big Brother" dispatched the PMO to pick up what was described as "an elderly gentleman in a yellow shirt."

When PMO arrived on scene, they found CDR Self trying to get his 20 miles in for the day and muttering something about the new Redskins mascot and Woodie Guthrie.

Confused by his ramblings, PMO had no choice but load him up and track down his chain of command.

The XO had no comment when approached for an interview by The Camel, and CDR Self just kept repeating "the universe is expanding, man."

Luckily the CMO was able to sleep through the night because we all know how he can get when he's up without his coffee. Plus LCDR Salazar gives him plenty to be concerned with.

If you know anyone who is old and long in the tooth, do not set them outside or to pasture. Never forget that they are people too that rate the same kind of dignity as most of us.

I think I Googled "dementia in the desert" for this pic

Probably what Dr. Self looked like in the desert before PMO snatched him up.

ROLE I SOLIDER EARNS SPECIAL LIBERTY AS JENGA CHAMPION

Specialist Vanessa Acosta needs to work a little less now that she is the NATO MMU Jenga champion.

Sergeant First Class Berthold has awarded the young solider a rare half-day of special liberty from normal working hours after winning the local Jenga championship held at the pharmacy compound.

Specialist Acosta was ecstatic to hear the news about only having to work a half-day.

"Yeah, 12 hours is half of a day," said the senior enlisted sea daddy.

Thirsty Camel beat writers captured the moment and said it best when they claimed that in a fierce series of three games, youth had the definitive advantage over the aging bones of her competitor.

Pronounced "Acoosta," as in 'cukoo bird,' the Role I war hero is accepting challenges.

"I used to run the beer pong table back home, but now I run the leaning tower of Jenga, come at me bro," was the only reprintable quote from the champion.

> ***"I used to run the beer pong table back home, but now I run the leaning tower of Jenga, come at me bro"***

SEA / SEL CALL THE SHORTEST IN HISTORY, LIKE THEMSELVES

Earlier today the top enlisted at Whiskey Rotation had a come to Jesus meeting with all of the bluejackets.

"I was expecting the Call to be like the 'moment of truth' in boot camp," said on directorate Leading Petty Officer.

In reality it was one of the shortest meetings in the history of having to get all dressed up for. Although the required threads was the OCP uniform, it has been uncovered that some things are only a formality.

"It was wasn't exactly locker room talk, but it wasn't exactly the state of the union either."

In the dire attempt for the most accurate account of the situation, it can summarized as follows:

"The reason why the meeting was so damn short was because of the continued investment the Chiefs have put into their Sailors. They are out there, on the deckplates, from their ivory towers and had the pulse of the enlisted staff well before anyone stepped into C-17."

Again, Definitely Not a Role 3 MMU Publication

THIRSTY CAMEL MAIL BAG

Dear Camel,

My name is Jesse. Huge fan, first time writer. I'm afraid that I am a candy-ass. What is best in life to be more like you? -Jesse, age 32

Hello Jesse,

I actually get this question more often than you may think. I try to crush my enemies, see them driven before me, and start each morning with a cup of CMO's coffee. Good luck out there, it's a jungle. Thanks for reaching out, always nice to meet a fan.

Camel,

I think you're a poser, and only try to be funny when other people are around. How does it feel to be the Carlos Mencia of the Whiskey Rotation? Signed "Jed"

Hey Asshat,

Just so you know, Joe Rogan probably has a better haircut than you. You try breaking out amongst a group of peers rather than sit in your dark hole and watch the world as it passes you by.

PSA FROM THE EDITORIAL STAFF

The writing staff at the Thirsty Camel needs to disclose that this publication is written strictly for the love of entertainment, and despite its most valiant attempts to the contrary, is not knowingly used for any professional gain in terms of Sailor recognition or ranking. Each Issue takes about 8 hours of time spent away from full-disclosure civic service such as the chapel. To wear the cloak of anonymity is a heavy crown to bear, but in a way it's perfect because that's what camels do. They are the unsung heroes when they put the team on their backs in the service & entertainment of others. So enjoy and happy reading!

CMO'S COFFEE EARNS PRESTIGIOUS CJOA-A 'CUP OF JOE" AWARD

Our gentlemanly CMO has a lot to smile about lately.

First, he was relieved to learn that the 'Biggest Loser' contest is about weight-loss and second, his refreshingly bold coffee, the product of an O6 level secret recipe and inspired technique, has won recognition from CJOA-A as a worthy 'Cup of Joe'.

Not only is this stalwart CAPT the first Whiskey Rotation representative to win the famed 'C-JOAA C'JOE' (FYSA that's pronounced C'JOE C'JOE, Senior Chief) label of approval, but he is the first Sailor ever to win any award for coffee in a Joint Command controlled by the Army.

The Thirsty Camel has learned that the long-standing bias of the Army against Navy coffee goes back generations from the moment when General MacArthur took a sip of Admiral Halsey's liquid creation and immediately cursed its deck-stripping capabilities.

MacArthur reportedly never drank coffee aboard ship again and was thereafter frequently heard bemoaning his foolishness for humoring Halsey's offer of a steaming cup.

'It is true that the Army has probably taken this coffee grudge too far,' stated an unnamed 4-Star on the 'Cup of Joe' judging panel, "but clearly it's time to let bygones be bygones."

"Coffee of this superiority cannot be ignored, even if a swabby produced it."

Stop by the CMO's office mid-morning and see if you agree. The Thirsty Camel certainly does! Before you do however, do not forget to give the proper greeting of the day, knock 3 three times and request permission to enter. CMO is an important fellow.

Chinaware teacup

Wardroom Coffee Cup

Seaman Timmy: Chief, is there something moving in your coffee?
Chief: Don't touch, it's perfect.

Enlisted Coffee

26 July 2020
Days 157, 158, 159 & 160

I'm unimpressed with myself that I have four pages to write, but I do not think I will be short on content. You see, today I was weak and felt sorry for myself. I really didn't do anything. The highlight of today was getting my haircut. Of course, it was the deployment special, a buzz cut low enough for a common onlooker to wonder if I enjoy *American History X* (2000) a little too much, if you pick up my drift. I've always enjoyed short hair unlike my two brothers.

Enough of that; the only other thing I did on my day off was buy a new tube for my bike. It popped last night. I completed a task Chief Melvin Atangan gave both HM2 Renardo Reid and me. In preparation for the hospital closing, we were tasked to find all wall hangings which could potentially be used against the United States government for propaganda purposes. Essentially, what we had to do was tag everything that put America in a good light because from an enemy perspective it could be used in a bad light.

What was most interesting was working with Renardo Reid. I can't remember if I mentioned it in Volume I of this journal, but I'm not the biggest Reid fan. It's easy to work with him professionally, but I'm not in a hurry to bury the hatchet with him. According to my roommate, that is exactly what he wanted to do, which I avoided at all costs. Kudos to Reid for wanting to be the bigger man if that was true.

That was all today, and yesterday there wasn't a big difference. I got home around 1000, was sleeping by 1100, and didn't wake up again until 2000. It felt amazing, and I'm very thankful to HM1 Wilson for reading the situation and getting me out of the base-wide mass casualty exercise. From what I heard he took some heat for making that decision, but what it created was a more loyal worker.

One may be wondering how or why I was so tired. It all stems back from two days ago when the second soldier within two weeks shot themselves in the head. Not only did this guy survive, unlike the first soul, but the bullet went straight up through his dome in such a way that he was able to open the door to his barracks, walk into the hospital, and place himself on the gurney. It was nothing short of amazing. Later on, I saw the droplets of blood on the blacktop to confirm that he walked.

When I got to the Emergency Room, he was responsive to pain and acted like he knew what the hell was going on. Then part one of the fun started. Of course, they put him under and intubated the guy. They got him stable enough for the CT scan where they found bleeding and pressure building in his skull. Well, duh. It was still so surreal because the exit wound was a small hole, and not a blow-out like what we see in the movies.

So, they rushed him to the Operating Room, and LCDR Deguzman, HM1 LaPenna, and I were on standby near the Operating Room. When it was my turn, I was asked if I wanted to scrub in. Not really scrub but put on the necessary protective equipment/garments. It was there I realized the operating room is the farthest thing from the pharmacy. The first thing I noticed was how bright it all was. The room smelled sterile. There were a number of people who were in the room, either working or observing as I was.

Dr. Jonathan Cooke, the neurosurgeon, was at the head and it's then I began to lose my appetite. This guy's skull, at least the frontal portion was gone. I saw his brain. It was wrapped in a natural casing, not giving its clear gray hue, but almost bluish. It was not pulsating. Doctor Cooke was rooting around where I'm assuming his sinus cavity was supposed to be.

I was told the main mission was to control the cranial pressure and stop the bleeding. They'd leave his skull off and replace it with a prosthetic later. After that he was sent to the Intensive Care Unit and that's when pharmacy went to work. By now it was me and LCDR Deguzman, and we worked for hours. Each taking turns in the hood. After he left at 2200, they came up with new meds almost regularly for every 90 minutes that I had to make. It sucked.

He was flown out at about 0630 that morning. I suppose there is more I could say about it, but for what purpose? My thoughts on suicide are not compassionate. This soldier thought he didn't want to live, but the lengths we went through to determine that he did are almost comical. If he does survive, and I'll never know, he'll be one limited individual. Maybe he'll be happy he's alive, but at what cost?

I'm almost done with my Wisconsin Olympian book, so that is good. Called my mom tonight. My honorary Aunt Shari was visiting for the weekend. The boys seemed super excited when I called. "Hi Papa!" always warms my heart. I'm already building some good content for the next *Thirsty Camel*, too.

I will never kill myself. That pain is mine.

Postscript: It doesn't get any more graphic than that. There are other published stories that speak to the gore of war, especially in a combat environment. This entry was my deployment. We saved an American life. Other guys I talked to who have been to the Role III hospital talked about the mass casualties and weary days of intensity. I never had my shot. Although I was there and was ready, my war stories are generally summarized in this one entry. The rest of this story was my journey through every other day, how I made it through, and the parts that are usually left on the editing room floor. I suppose what is most unique about my experience at the KAF Role III was that it was the last rotation at the longest serving combat hospital, and we worked through the COVID-era. Although I would gladly accept my garrison cap at the local VFW one day, I'm not one to brag that I was on a "real deployment." Maybe something to work through one day.

27 July 2020
Day 161

And the hits just keep on coming. Today was another day bent over the barrel. We had a helicopter crash. The first guy who came in was burnt up and had multiple fractures to his arm. We were working full tilt all day long. HM1 LaPenna, who I relieved, didn't go home until 1930. The day just flew by.

The second patient of the day had another head injury leading him to have a craniotomy. Although I wasn't in the Operating Room for this guy, I know part of his skull is missing.

It was Mail Call today and it was a good day. HM2 Mario Torres had a package sent to me. It was filled with treats from Japan. Fun fact, it was the first care package sent from Japan besides my family. So yes, I'm a little surprised by that. Who knows, maybe it's in the mail. Coffee came in today, another 5 lb bag from Enderley Coffee Company, but a different flavor than last time.

After the smoke settled a bit, I tried to change my bike tire, but couldn't do it myself. HM2 Jesse John helped me out big time. Will probably still buy a new bike, although I saw on the tire the max weight limit was 198 lb. Oops!

Watched most of *Indiana Jones and the Last Crusade* (1989), too. It was action packed and charming. It's just hard to explain how busy I was. Oh, I got an email from Aunt Laura. I guess self-publish?

Postscript: A majority of our casualties were not American. Instead, they were Afghani. All of these patients were given a pseudonym to keep their identity a secret. They were given different names depending on the admin department's mood. Sometimes they were given Star Wars characters, but towards the end, the Executive Officer (XO) wanted to keep them all whiskey brands to keep continuity with our rotation namesake.

28 July 2020
Day 162

On second thought, after much deliberation, I will make an entry for today. Originally, I did not believe that there was much to be said about today, but it would be problematic in a couple of areas. First, it is my goal to capture every day's events, and unless I can help it, to get away from grouping. In other words, I must force myself to write even if I don't feel like it.

Second, enough minor details occurred that would otherwise be lost to history should I group my days. That would be a disservice to the entire project. I ordered three books on how to self-publish. They were mailed to Japan for my return.

Chief AT's notes came back on my Sailor of the Month write-up. It was disheartening to read at times, because the reality of my life is two competent First Classes in my shop and others who I'm objectively ranked against are placed in positions of leadership by virtues of right time, right place. It's just frustrating and a common theme in my professional life of not having a shot at failing.

Started a new book on loan from HM1 Wilson called *Stillness is the Key.* So far I'm digging it. LCDR Deguzman took no less than three hours creating an online customs label. Man has half the alphabet after his name and still struggles with technology.

Took a long nap, but not before calling home and talking for half an hour. Bathroom is gutted, very happy to see the progress.

Postscript: "Having a shot at failing." I would often compare my path to Rocky Balboa. He just wanted to go the distance. In order to see if he could go the distance, he was given a shot. Had Apollo Creed never plucked him from obscurity and given him his shot, we would never know if he would fail or succeed. The key was he was given a shot. I don't like saying given a chance at succeeding because to me that sounds too cliche, and if I'm going to fail, I'll probably learn something. The second part of that was that Saori was already using our "deployment money" to remodel our bathroom.

29 July 2020
Day 163

Happy birthday cousin JJ! If I had actually sat down to wonder whose birthday it really was, I'm sure that I would have remembered, but Facebook was for once useful.

My hands feel like hamburger meat today because I went lifting with LT Scott Byrd. It was more farmer carries than anything. I did surprise myself though that all together I deadlift over 300 lb, but it was like 155 lb in each hand, and I'd walk 15 yards or so and turn around. Tomorrow will no doubt be a different story on how I feel.

Time spent on the treadmill before working out left more to be desired. I only burned 250 calories and was on for less than 15 minutes. The calves just weren't having it. Only a couple of days and I'll be back at it like old times. I'm chasing 30 minutes straight as my next goal.

Besides that, it was my day off. Woke up at 1000, putted around the room, called Saori; she just had her haircut and looked beautiful as ever. Oh, when I called the boys at their bedtime, Josey took the phone and showed me the gutted bathroom. First, he spoke in Japanese, but I told him to speak English. He then said the bathroom was broken. I almost cried right then. Can't wait for more experiences like that.

I deleted Instagram late last night and finished Issue #9 of *The Thirsty Camel*, too.

Postscript: Maybe a lot of parents take for granted being able to talk to their kids, or, more specific to me, to have their kids talk to them. Josiah up to this point could understand most of what I said when I tried to talk how I would to any 5-year-old, but his output of communication often left for quiet conversations. He is slowly coming around, but his primary language is Japanese. This only motivates me to learn the language more, but I still talk to him in English because besides his mother and grandparents back in Wisconsin, his only inlet to English is the cartoons I put on for him. Listening to Josey and Atticus speak in Japanese to one another though is so endearing, probably because I just love seeing them be brothers to one another.

Definitely Not a Role 3 MMU Publication

The Thirsty Camel

Issue IX

Roll-out Date Not Important, Like the Morale

Special points of interest:

- It started as a kiss how could it end up like this?
- Is this the real life, or is it just fantasy?
- I know the pieces fit 'cause I watched them fall away.
- Sitting at a corner in Winslow, AZ.
- Cookies are now a non-formulary item in the pharmacy: BANNED!

Inside this issue:

Directors Rumble	2
Help Our Own	2
Friday Corpsman	2
Trade Demands	3
Bad Boyz For Life	3
LT's Called Up	3
COTs Love Life	4
Tip The Real Ones	4
Bored Surgeons	4

BUNKER BOMBER DISCOVERS TIME TRAVEL

LT Wilcox found his roommate LT Veatch so frustratingly older and wiser over the month of July that he finally sat him down for a battle buddy chat, asking, "What the doo-hickey is going on with you lately, roomie?" (Apparently 'doo-hickey' is the only curse word that LT Wilcox knows.)

His fellow OR Nurse, at first reluctant, faded under Wilcox's irritatingly amiable probing. On the 4th of July, LT explained, during his daily bunker search, he was entranced by an image reminding him of a Civil War battle that occurred on the beautiful farmland of Kentucky in 1862.

(FYSA, the dedicated LT combs bunker walls for inspiration to share with his soggy-minded shipmates. 'You have to dumb it down for them. They wouldn't know a Jackson Pollock from a Thomas Kinkaid," he has told his wife.)

The LT, enthralled by the shimmering image, lightly brushed it with his hand and was immediately transported to a fence row in Old Kentucky sporting a gleaming image of a Predator taking off from KAF.

The LT says he spent the next 3 years assisting in surgery in a variety of campaigns culminating in his witnessing of the meeting of Grant and Lee at Appomattox.

'Holy Scrapple!' shouted LT Wilcox. "That is so cool! You have got to take me with you next time!"

LT Veatch, however, is not so eager. "I'm a changed man. I've been to Hell and back and it ain't just for fun."

For now, The Thirsty Camel recommends that Whiskey shipmates give LT Veatch some latitude and allow him his time ruminating on the works of Kafka, Dumas, and Hemingway.

"How did you get home?" the Thirsty Camel inquired.

"I hitched a ride with some Johnnies back to Kentucky and found that shining Predator image," he matter-of-factly replied.

"Where else, that is, when and where else would you like to go?" we asked.

"Maybe with John Paul Jones aboard the Bonhomme Richard, the original not the infamous," he mused with a faraway look in his eye.

THIRSTY CAMEL GOING PAPERLESS

The Camel is a team player. It's pro-green and on the cutting edge of environmental preservation. In many ways the Camel sees itself as the Theodore Roosevelt of its generation.

What the Camel is also acutely aware of is who signs their performance evaluation.

From this day to the last, the Thirsty Camel will now go paperless.

There are real concerns that the general doesn't have a sense of humor, and we are in no hurry of testing that theory.

Lots of leaders sell souls to the Night King in exchange for reaching flag rank, but that is absolute speculation.

In the meantime, cheers to hanging onto the morale we have left.

DIRECTORS RUMBLE OVER LT BYRD'S "OFFICE"

In a tell-all memorandum, the most unimportant important staff member of Whiskey Rotation is under fire for leaking highly confidential information from the last Board of Directors, or BOD, meeting.

"What LT Hollins did to us is nothing compared what we are going to do to him," quoted one pissed off leader.

Another officer concurred with the pain felt around the highest echelons of Role 3 leadership with one director of the cage-fighting persuasion hinting that Edward Snowden was a joke compared to this loss of trust.

Benedict Hollins

In the memorandum from the first man to be voted off of Important Island, it was argued who will assume LT Byrd's shithole office.

There has been a lot of chatter about some senior officers not having their own office while this lowly lieutenant does.

Of course the PME office is off-limits and for good measure. LT Quinn protects her den more fiercely than a honey badger. There are some things in this world not dying over.

LT Byrd's office, different story. In spite of the department head's proven track record of promotable qualities, the tiny closet in which he harbors his care packages is in line to be snatched up by someone else.

"RIIP," but the rumble over the real estate should be epic to see. LT Hollins was not available to comment.

DR WARNER IS LOSING GAINS, AND MIND TOO

Crises come in different forms and each one is projected a bit differently from person to person.

LT Gerrid Warner is in the midst of such a complex. According to a letter sent to the Thirsty Camel editor outlining the pickle he is currently finding himself in.

"Bro, I'm losing these gains and it's consuming my mind too."

Consumption has taken too many spirits, just ask Edgar Allan Poe, but we can't have our counter-balance to LT Reeder down for the count.

"Bro, I'm losing these gains and it's consuming my mind too."

Too many things are left to be tolerated, just ask anyone feeling the recent loss of all the stress outlets , but we need to band together and get LT's gains back.

Maybe if ED played nicer with ICU, LT could be turned back into a pretzel by some good ol boy Dept Heads.

PETTY OFFICER PARCHMON FIRED ON DAY OFF

HM2 Parchmon had some explaining to do to his mentor yesterday as he was apparently fired on his day off.

"Every time I'm in the kitchen, you're in the kitchen."

According to sources, the leading petty officer of the emergency department was relieved of duty as the simulation lab director when six rotations worth of clothing was mysteriously thrown away. The dummies will now be forever "trauma naked" thanks to HM2's lack of protection of all government property in view.

HM2's face when he heard the news

Violation of the 1st General Order of a Sentry is punishable up to death, so in some circles, he's getting off light.

LT HOWELL DEMANDS A TRADE TO DAYS

Lieutenant Ed Howell is not a happy camper. Reports have been confirmed that he has spoken through his agent that he is not satisfied working on nights, but for a rather peculiar reason.

"I'm getting fat working with LCDR Bansil, all she does is make me sit in a corner and feed me all kinds of delicious food."

The night crew, where the suppression of melancholy turned into a daily occurrence.

LT Howell's self-portrait

When bringing the matter up to the ICU Department Head, it was said that he as first laughed at, told to shut the f@ck up, and told, "this is the way."

The trade demand is not going over well with the Reservist Nursing Union either.

Union President LCDR Rachel Petrus, "This is a huge unbalance to nursing bargaining agreement we signed when we got our fat signing bonus. LT Howell's request is not in alignment with our values."

With so many patients to shepherd at night these days, there is no difference between light and day. It's getting into LT Howell's "git some" sessions at Swole 3. It is strongly rumored that Mr. Howell just wants to lift with Dr. Warner again.

Hang in there LT, just vent your worries to your roommate like a couple of OR nurses we all know.

HOLLINS AND WINK: BAD BOYZ FOR LIFE

LT Hollins and Senior Chief Wink have new monikers as the Bad Boyz of Whiskey Rotation.

As hilarious it would be for the day to cite a story about a couple of yahoo drunk drivers, bombing around a warzone at 12mph, this is not that day.

In fact, this is a story about the kindness and generosity of the First Class Petty Officer Mess, coming together to support their Senior Enlisted Advisor.

"I appreciate the First Classes for stepping up and graciously donating their vehicle to their fearless leader."

"I appreciate the First Classes for stepping up and donating their vehicle to their fearless leader."

It's true, while one vehicle was impounded for flippantly defying the general's rules, another was used in the effort to walk less... and make base-wide meetings.

As for LT Hollins, well, he got a consolation mustache ride from HM2 Terrell.

TAYLOR AND DOWNEY CALLED UP FROM MINORS

In a game-time call, the Executive Officer made a call down to the nursing bullpen to call up Lieutenants Greg Downey and Michele Taylor from night shift to work on the day crew.

This pic was hard to find. Manager tapping his forearm to call in the bullpen.

XO making the call

"It wasn't an easy call, but I wanted youth injected in the lineup of veterans we already got," said the Levi Garret fan.

Historically a switch like this is not rare to see. Lots of XO's shake up the lineup mid-deployment in order to instill a fiery spirit from the days of training.

Although the stats of Downey and Taylor are nothing to so special they need to write home about, the front office is excited to evaluate the budding talent for the rest of the season.

[This space reserved for all the Corpsmen who picked up off the test @ Role III]

ROLE 3 SURGEONS BORED

When CDR Cooke passed his kidney stone's he "was so high he could have passed a porcupine backwards and wouldn't have felt a thing." There are Thirsty Camels and thirsty surgeons. The latter have been so bored they took the passed stones and operated on them because there has been nothing else to do. The samples were sent to the lab as if they weren't buried in enough PCRs. During these tumultuous times, at the apex of self-entertainment, we will look to the surgeons who will make the most of any opportunity. May we stand on their shoulders.

SEND SOME LOVE TO THE JANITORIAL STAFF & BEYOND

Far too often the janitorial staff are the unsung heroes of the Role 3 MMU building. They are here literally 24 hours a day, and their customer service puts even the best trained American to shame.

Any person who cleans up after CDR Self is a rare breed, and they do it day in and day out.

Then there is the other contractors in the building. CIO is only a position, but who is the real genius behind the scenes? SUPPO can't even get toilet paper, but Sean and the boys over at MEDLOG are the ones delivering the narcotics LT Warner so eagerly tries to acquire.

The Sailors along for the ride are mere placeholders to the real movers and shakers here. We tip our hats to you all. The work does not go unnoticed by the Camel.

Scrubs Janitor here. Had to find a relatable pic that we could all bond with. #medical #comedy

CHIEF OF TRAUMA DATED JANIS JOPLIN

Some stories to not belong to Hollywood. They in fact belong to the stars. This story is about the volatile love between Whiskey's Chief of Trauma and legendary rocker Janis Joplin.

It all started when COT was living a rebel life in San Francisco. He had just left the Montana farm and really embraced the Haight-Ashbury district culture.

One rainy day he glazed his way into the Stardust Lounge when he saw an up and coming musician solo on the mic.

The legend is said that Kris Kristofferson was away in the head when COT confidently walked up to the muse and swept her off her feet in the middle of the set.

Like King Kong with his prize, they ran off into the Red Wood forest where they lived in the trees talking about the meanings to life and the sound of one hand clapping.

But the future doc could not sustain the free lifestyle, and had finally come up to his senses. He had to leave, and the broken-hearted girl was truly devastated.

Before COT rode off into the sunset on his Vespa, they shared one last "California Cigarette" when she ran back inside to write both "Me and Bobby McGee" (COT's pseudonym while in the woods) and "Piece of My Heart" in memoriam of their time together.

On a sweltering night, we can still hear soft cries from the office. That's how the Camel heard it!

LT Dan circa 1984.

COT AS A YOUNG MAN

Stock photo of Janis Joplin smoking a "cigarette"

JANIS, STAR-CROSSED LOVER

ICU NURSES

There is a little "boot" in all of us at any given time. It does not matter if you are the saltiest Master Chief or the heavily-hazed Seamen Recruit, if you are unfamiliar with something, you're setting yourself up to be educated. Sometimes that education is painless, and sometimes it will be written about in a book. My education with nurses, especially those in the intensive care unit, is one of those latter experiences.

My career history in the Navy has been essentially overseas clinics. Most notably in Japan under the command of US Naval Hospital Yokosuka. It's true; out of my four permanent duty stations so far, three of them have been at branch clinics in Japan. We like to call US Naval Hospital (USNH) Yokosuka the "mothership," "core," or "enterprise" among the clinics. My lone non-Japan command was the USS Theodore Roosevelt (CVN-71) in Norfolk, VA. My experiences on the ship will spring up in other places, but for now we are talking about nurses in a non-operational setting.

To be a nurse in the Navy, you need to have your Bachelor of Science in nursing (BSN). Nurses are officers and proud ones at that. I would think they are proud because they come in at the very bottom of the Officer pay scale as an 0-1, or Ensign. This is a rank where Dr. Seuss and Tim Burton would thrive. It is a bizarre place because you are an officer, yet no one takes you seriously. There are of course the occasional unicorns we call "mustangs" who have previous enlisted experience, but by and large, they enter the workforce at 22 to 24 years old and as an officer there is plenty to be responsible for. This is rich because they sometimes have trouble being responsible for themselves. Fraternization is rampant at this pay grade and many enlisted Sailors have earned their "O" qualification through the naivete of the most junior officers. They have trouble knowing how to "Navy" and are learning how to do their job at the same time. The amount of shit they must eat their first couple of years in the service gives them an edge which is unmistakable, and for the most part that edge is carried with them for the rest of their careers.

Then there is me at the branch clinics. The enlisted medical force, or Hospital Corpsmen, are the workhorses of the operation. Nurses are important, they have their place, but I never saw a nurse give an enema, apply a scrotum saddle, or insert a foley catheter. That is the Corpsman's job. Nurses at the clinics assume a much more administrative intensive role, and that is fine. From my perspective and my own experiences, they were never actually boots on ground unless things turned sideways, which almost never happened. This all changed in Afghanistan.

Most of the officers were reservists. They had real jobs back home and the concept of a Corpsman is not generally practiced let alone utilized. In the Navy, if working with active-duty service men and women, a Hospital Corpsman has a lot of autonomy on how much medical care they can render. To an outsider this can be frightening to think about, and as a result I will stay quieter than I normally would on how high, wide, and deep we can go in the service of our country. It did not, however, change the perception I had on nurses being essentially desk jockeys, and how my world was rocked in the best of ways.

We had lieutenants changing colostomy bags, wiping butts, changing bed sheets, doing all the best kinds of work that would normally be so far away from their paygrade it was hard to watch. Although I couldn't help but crack a smile and sigh with relief that they were doing the work and not me, I couldn't help except to prepare to be told to change out a wound dressing each time I delivered an IV bag of fentanyl. That day never came.

The nurses in the intensive care unit did it all, and as much as they were chatty about their working conditions, they made a pretty strong argument for their cause, especially looking back on what they did. We had no electronic charting, it was all done with paper, and they were on top of their game. There was no rest for the weary, they pulled their weight and I know for a fact they kept some patients alive through some of the darkest of hours. I know this because I was there to deliver their medications, always waiting to be told to roll up my sleeves and join them.

There were of course other nurses at the hospital, notably the emergency room and operation room, and they earned their paychecks too, but the ICU nurses at Whiskey Rotation get the articles written about them. Going from being a nurse practitioner as a civilian to wiping the ass of a bullet-riddled patient as a reservist had to be a humbling experience, but by and large they were professionals who tried their best with what they had. They definitely showed me another side of nursing in Navy medicine, and I'm proud to have worked with so many great people. For the record, if any of our enlisted folk earned their "O" qualification, it was never proven and will remain lost to history and would forever stay in the desert.

31 July 2020
Days 164 & 165

It might be me, but the evenings might be getting cooler. What is probably happening is, I'm being more tolerant of my circumstances, but as I sit outside waiting for my laundry to dry at the self-service, I can't help but notice how it's not absolutely miserable. Possibly the turning of the page, but who knows.

I read in the published minutes of the most recent Board of Directors meeting that X-Ray Rotation begins their pipeline in Norfolk on Monday (it's Friday today, according to my watch). This of course is great news, and HM3 Wes Alden predicts just 25 more duty days. With a duty day every three days, we're on the same shift, roughly 75 days to go. I don't think I'll tell Saori just yet because I don't want to get her hopes up.

Everything is still so fluid. Yesterday I bought a bike for $60. I'm horrible at haggling so it was "sticker price." Only three months old, it's a dream compared to the piece of crap I was riding. The only bummer about my new bike is that it's short on bells and whistles. No light or rack in the back. Brakes are a little splashy, but I can hopefully change that soon enough.

The two Afghan men involved in the helicopter crash are still admitted, and no release date is expected soon. The one patient with brain damage is keeping us particularly busy in the pharmacy, but that's also why we are here.

I was daydreaming today about missing out on essentially all of Saori's pregnancy with Winston. How I wasn't there to feel her belly or lift heavy things for her. You know, just being around. It made me sad, wiped a mental tear, and went back to work. It's the only thing I could do.

The reason why I didn't write last night was because I was too upset, and I don't know why. HM1 Wilson took the speaker in the pharmacy outside to lift with his friends. I was working. Anyway, it was eating at me, and I popped off. He was of course pissed right back, but refrained from beating the sass out of me, calmed down, we spoke normally about it, and went along with our day. Either way, it wasn't about the stupid speaker, but I don't know what it was.

Was a good couple of days on the treadmill. Yesterday was a new personal record for straight run time at 30:00 at 5.0 speed. I have now increased starting speed to 5.1 and will increase by 0.1 every successful five-minute increment without stopping. Today I set a new 60:00 distance and calorie personal record. Old was 4.65 miles and 1,132 calories. Today was 4.79 miles and 1,157 calories. I should probably be weighing myself sooner than later. Probably next post duty morning.

Sailor in the Spotlight articles are done for *The Whiskey Ration.*

Postscript: The Whiskey Ration *is the name of the official command newsletter. It was brought up before but deserves a refresher. It was now fun looking for the official stories to write and delegate responsibilities. More on that later. The speaker story may have been the start of our end. Not like a crash and burn, but we only spent all of our time with the same people. My life was within a two-square-kilometer area. I could be seen at the barracks, hospital, chow hall, laundry mat, Navy Exchange store, or on my way to one of those places. We had no 24-hour indoor gym, the basketball court and team sports were closed, too. We didn't have a Morale, Welfare, Recreation (MWR), USO, or recreation outlets outside of these places. Luckily, I liked to read and write, and if I liked spending up to two hours a day at Swole 3, I could gather around a bench press with everyone else. So yes, by this time I was miserable.*

1 Aug 2020
Day 166

Already August. Time is passing by quickly, especially when you look back. If we look too far into the future, time can get overwhelming. On the other hand, when I look back to the beginning, I can feel a little sad. I feel that way because I ask myself just what I accomplished, and more importantly what I have to show for it.

When I look back in general it's not a whole lot done, but if I were to break it down, I think there is a good deal. I need to allow myself permission to cherish the victories where I can get them.

Today was my day off, but I was at the hospital for 10 hours. Started at noon, but to be fair there was a bonfire held by the MWR Committee. Couple of things here. One, it was interesting to see everyone in a looser environment. Second, because I feel better about myself and the way I look I was able to talk myself into enjoying the gathering. That is one positive I'm taking with me.

This time of the month is always a busy time for the pharmacy because there is a lot of turnover with expiration checks and squaring away the books for the Controlled Substance Inventory Board. As much as I wanted to work on other projects, for a time all three techs were in there working.

Wasn't feeling it on the treadmill today, but still climbed on.

Postscript: I loved the Controlled Substance Inventory Board, or CSIB. They are supposed to be an independent team that comes to the pharmacy to audit the history of our controlled medications. Because this is not their primary job, they need help from the pharmacy to help ensure the books are straight. Well, we begin our assistance well before they arrive. When there was a discrepancy with the logs, I felt like I was always the short straw to figure out why. This could be a ridiculously long process. Sometimes because I was so inexperienced with doing this, and other times in our haste mistakes were made and you had to explain why. Sometimes it was my fault, sometimes I was lucky. Either way, I was always proud of myself for finding the answers to that month's riddle.

3 Aug 2020
Day 167 & 168

Some good stuff in the past couple of days. The reason why I didn't write last night was because I had a robust debate with Dr. Christina "Dearest" Solomon over a great many things that I don't typically get to talk about while in the Navy. There's never a bad conversation with her, and last night was no different. I don't think she liked to hear that once she found the person she was meant to be with, how much it would dramatically change the dynamic of our friendship. To me, there is nothing wrong with that because it's life.

Today was Mail Call. The only piece of mail was from the phantom post cardist. To be fair, snail mail for Victor Rotation is still trickling in like today. But this same person has consistently produced a postcard every week. All I know is the card comes out of Milwaukee and they quote Theodore Roosevelt.

Probably the biggest news is the FRAGO, or Fragmented Order, about our future. Because no one else will read this until after the fact, I'm not concerned with Operational Security, or OPSEC. Anyway, there is a real possibility we will not be here to see the start of October. There are a couple of layers, but the second-best news is they are keeping this building and we won't be moving to another location. Again, still nothing to really tell Saori until it's even more clear. It's still all the buzz amongst the people tonight.

I worked out with LT Byrd tonight, and he introduced me to atlas stones. Not totally against them but will take some getting used to. I had the 115 lb stone and he was rocking the 175 lb rock. After dropping the stone, I actually got dizzy and needed to sit down. That's a mark of a good job, right?

Yesterday, the biggest news to come from the day might have been Saori and I had to reconvene the naming commission. The fact I reneged on Winston would not have bothered Saori, but when I told her that my mother wasn't necessarily onboard, back to the starting point we went. We agreed on two things. The first was I submitted my final four names, and we would not disclose until the kid came to greet the world.

HM2 Chris Parchmon wants to put me up for Motivator of the Month for *The Whiskey Ration* newsletter. I had some hesitation with this, but after talking to Captain Daniel Kahler I learned about accepting gifts with grace. There is something to be said about allowing someone the chance to try to do something nice for another because sometimes gifts are not actually about the recipient at all.

Postscript: Since my return from the deployment, the "accepting gifts with grace" story has possibly been my most cited learning experience to younger Sailors. Maybe it was CAPT Kahler's delivery, or it was what I needed to hear most at that time. Either way, it has stuck with me. There were plans at the time to move the hospital to another building. Because the Role III hospital was so close to the airfield, we would move closer inboard as the base continued to shrink. Luckily for Whiskey Rotation, we didn't have to move. I remember being on the USS Theodore Roosevelt (CVN-71) coming out of the Refuel Complex Over Haul (RCOH) and moving a tiny pharmacy. That was a terrible time. Moving all of the medications, equipment, and supplies down the road would have taken an entire week. They made the right call.

8 Aug 2020
Day 169, 170, 171, 172 & 173

These past five days are a perfect example of time flying by. I honestly had enough to say every day, but for one reason or another I let the moment pass. Before I knew it, I'm five days late. Looking back on it, I'm almost amazed at how quick a moment comes and goes. Anyway, all that jazz brings us neatly to where we are now, and we will start with today because in a selfish way it is the most important.

At about 0900, the Skipper announced the winners to July's Sailor of the Month. Of the Second Classes, I was among three other candidates. My board performance was strong, but not spectacular. The board believed I was the winner, and the Captain endorsed their recommendation. It was a bit surreal; I felt the same buzz from when I was meritoriously promoted on the ship back in 2012. I honestly can only remember feeling relieved when the Sailor of the Year was announced in Iwakuni back in 2016. In a way it felt like this was a long time coming. The moment was building and building. All my late nights and long days seemed to have (finally) paid off. Many hours were spent at the office "when I was not supposed to be there," grinding and working on either this or that. Helping where I could and trying my hardest at what I did. This does not mean the other nominees gave up or put in minimal effort. Like the Rock would say, no one is going to out work me, and that's what I feel like I did.

Of course, it was not without help. HM1 LaPenna and HM1 Wilson were on the board, but I think it was more of how they helped over not just the month, but since February. So then, where does it go from here? I worked really hard to climb this mountain and I want to stay on top of it. Until they say any different, I'm going to work toward going back-to-back Sailor of the Month. Is it selfish? Is it egomaniacal? Probably some of both, but I'm going to prove to myself that I'm not only the hardest working man in Sasebo, but on this deployment too. Yes, I am still swelled with confidence, but I would rather be like this than not wanting to step up and seize my moment. How badly I wanted to forward the CO's email to my Chiefs back in Sasebo being like, "See?!" I refrained, and instead forwarded to Yani, Wydra, and a few of the kids.

Speaking of kids, Atticus was so naughty on the phone today! Had I been there I would have whooped his little ass the way he was sassing his mom and hitting her. That boy is in for a rude surprise if he keeps that up when I get home. Actually, he'll do it once and learn a hard lesson. Both Saori and I agree that Josiah will be a very good big brother whereas Atti will struggle adjusting to no longer being the baby.

Oh! The bathroom looks really good. Saori is sending pics and videos of the progress. The sink and cupboards are being installed after the Obon holiday, but they are able to bathe now which is good. The washer apparently broke and instead of $100 to fix the problem, Saori and her mom would rather spend $1,000 for a brand-new unit. Translation, no new bedroom set when I get home. Oh well, I am still not sure when or how I'll get the old dresser out of the house and the new one in at the moment.

Because we are talking about coming home, now is as good a time as ever to talk about the other latest and greatest news. The end is near, like a lot nearer than originally planned. It has been announced that the Army will be relieving Whiskey Rotation, and the day of the Role III Multinational Medical Unit will at last come to pass. The base is shrinking, and everything is becoming downgraded, including the medical capabilities. From a Role III that includes a brain surgeon and internal medicine physician to a Role II consisting of what I heard was 10 people.

I don't know what will happen to the pharmacy, and truth be told, I care less than I should. On one hand I was looking forward to handing off a pristine pharmacy, one that we, or HM1 LaPenna specifically, has spent weeks cultivating into a well-oiled machine, but the reality is I don't even know if the Role II will even have a pharmacy component. Who will close it out and what will happen to it remains an honest mystery as I write this.

Then there is the whole getting back home part. I just heard tonight from HM3 Wes Alden that we should be back to our parent commands by September 23, give or take a day. I guess Alden heard it from Senior Chief Wink that we're flying out either on Sept. 16 or 17. Are we going to Germany? Qatar? Who knows, but I do know I will enjoy reading this passage after the fact when I know how it really turns out. Until then, I better start mailing even more stuff home.

The two patients that were involved in the helicopter crash are still here. Although the brain guy is not trying to actively die in the past day or two, his schedule of meds has us up at weird hours making it in the hood.

There will come a time, however, that we will run out of medication for brain guy, an Afghan man we have been calling Sho Hungary. Say that again and consider the sense of humor the admin department has.

When they are stable enough to be transferred out, no doubt they will, and it's another rumor that we won't be accepting any new Afghan national patients. How nice that would be since a lion's share of our total patient load has not been Americans.

Still reading my book that HM1 Wilson recommended. Honestly, the last time I cracked it open was probably the same day as my last journal entry, but I don't know for sure.

What I have been allowing myself to do, however, is start to watch more movies. I took HM1 LaPenna's recommendation and watched *Empire Records* (1995). A young Liv Tyler can never go wrong. I also watched a Kevin Spacey movie from 2011 called *Margin Call* (2011). It's been in my queue for quite some time and I'm thankful that I finally got around to it.

After all these pages, I still enjoy journaling. I doubt I will continue as steadily as I am now, but I'm proud of myself for committing to this project. One day someone besides me will hopefully read and appreciate it.

Postscript: There is a lot to unpack here. Of the content left on the editing room floor, was my thoughts on my chain of command at Navy Medicine Readiness and Training Unit Sasebo, Japan. To wrap it nicely, a break was needed in the relationship, and this deployment was what the doctor ordered. The Sailor of the Month was a great vindication. "We don't want Rastall to go, we want [a different Sailor] instead." "For reading so much, you aren't very smart." Having a request chit denied to attend my wife's IVF insertion procedure. The list could go on, but succeeding in Role III only validated my self-worth, which, if anyone noticed in these pages, had been crippling. Hearing the news about our departure is the second-best day of any deployed service member's deployment. The best day is actually leaving.

14 Aug 2020
Day 174, 175, 176, 177, 178 & 179

There is something to be said about the stillness of the night. It's a feeling that ever since I was a boy, I have held in the highest of regards. I can't recall where it comes from, but for as long as I have been working, I have wanted to work the night shift.

To be fair, I write that without ever having to work nights, something I'm sure has taken years off the lives of both my uncles and brother-in-law. I remember driving at night with my Uncle George during some very impressionable years, my first semester at UW-Green Bay for starters. It was him who moved me from Baraboo to Green Bay, and it was done in the cover of night. Although too much time has come to pass to remember many conversations, I remember his selfless act to help his nephew. It was Uncle George who picked me up on the way to Two Harbors, MN, for one Easter where we met most of my family, but it was him who went out of his way to help a kid who knew nothing about anything. The song "Radar Love" by Golden Earring remains my favorite "night driving" song because of him.

So why share all of this? I'm writing in the middle of the night of course, and I feel at home doing it.

There has been a big wave that has been sweeping this deployment. In many regards it has brought joy, humility, and a much-needed reassurance. On the other hand, I am working through doubt, insecurity, and angst. As mentioned earlier, I won the Sailor of the Month award. What happened a couple of days later was the nominations came out for the Motivator of the Month, a separate recognition award. All nominations were for me except for my own vote, for a successful Third Class named Aubrie Lopez. I knew a peer, HM2 Chris Parchmon, led the campaign, and that was a high enough honor being recognized by a peer, but the number of personalized nominations really put it over.

Of course, I had to show humility and present a stoic performance and told LCDR Fitzgerald, the Public Affairs Officer that if it was anyone else, I would give the same recommendation; that no single Sailor should take up so much ink on a single issue of *The Whiskey Ration* newsletter. She told me she heard my advice, but it's her newsletter and I'm being put up for both recognitions. I told her that I'll sleep well knowing I gave the best recommendation I could.

Riding that wave was not enough though because I continued putting in the hours at work. HM2 Anthony Roberts came up to the pharmacy window and asked why I'm always working. I couldn't give him a good answer, just that I wasn't tired, I was inspired. Every Sailor would not have blamed me had I let off the gas. Afterall, I "made it."

In one weary moment I had asked LCDR Deguzman why I don't leave work when I don't have to be there. He said that it gets noticed who cuts out when they can and who stays to grind. That only stoked my fire, and as a result I have completed my second Green Belt project. This means a lot.

Before arriving in Sasebo in 2017, I told myself that I wanted to go to the green belt class and learn the science of process improvement. It meant a lot to me, and I placed taking that class as one of my top three reasons to stay in the Navy. I remember that before I met Chief Matt Struble, I was hellbent on separating in April 2020. This qualification was not easy, and I had definite help from LCDR Deguzman. It took extra time away from doing fun stuff such as reading, writing, and watching movies. Because I have attained this qualification, I could argue with my soul that this deployment was worth it to me. Of course, an end of tour award, or EOT, would be cool, too, but I will get to that in a moment.

I also had a satisfying conversation with HM2 Jesse John. I always enjoy talking to him and one regret is I didn't do it more often. We talked for literally hours, and it felt wholesome the entire time.

Then there was everything else to think about. Issue #10 of *The Thirsty Camel* was written and published. It was a good one I felt. The time stamp when published was 0300. The next morning, or afternoon rather, HM1 Wilson directed me to not write the *Camel* on government computers.

When I asked what was the article that did it, he shared that LCDR Deguzman wants me to be working on work when I'm at work. Okay, this explanation is a gift, and I understand that no one, especially a hospital director and Commander-select, needs to explain themselves to an E-5. Secondly, I almost felt joy because it was one less thing to have to work on. There is almost a bigger kick out of telling folks that I'm banned and seeing the looks on their faces than fighting this. The only thing I'm disappointed about is in Issue #10 I specifically said there was one final issue to be written that will now never happen.

As strange as that all was, it does not compare to the anxiety evaluations are bringing upon me. Technically mine is submitted, but I had to do a couple rewrites today. Why it came to me, and not my LPO, HM1 LaPenna, is between HM1 Wilson and him. I did what I was asked. Of course, I was not happy with some of the decisions. A complete line was crossed out, and instead of filling it in with something else, I left it blank. There was no guidance on what to put instead. The second heartache was having to change Sailor of the Month from two wins to one. HM1 Wilson's reasoning was that a) he wasn't certain there'd be an August Sailor of the Month and b) he's considering putting up a Sailor from radiology. That means either LPO HM2 Rexroat or HM2 Rodriguez. I like both, but I'm also competitive and feel like the most deserving Sailor should be recognized and not a "spread the wealth" mentality. Those who are killing it ought to have the first chance at glory. After all, it pays to be a winner. This will all become funny if I walk out of here as the #1 early-promote ranked Second Class, but I'm not hedging my bets if there is an opportunity to excel.

There is nothing else for me to do here except work. I want a dividend on the investment. We had a "redeployment" class with Senior Chief Wink. The class was mandatory, but interesting. Things to consider as we reintegrate with the rest of society.

I'm also packing up as much as I can because the post office on base is closing on the last day of August. My goal is to leave here with one seabag with my personal stuff only and my carry-on backpack.

We heard a nice rumor that there is a possibility we will depart from Role III in Qatar to head home. That will be the best possible situation, but although it came from Senior Chief Wink, there are many forces above us that can make a different decision. Plan for the worst and hope for the best.

Oh! Because I'm not an LPO, I was uninvited to the E-4 Evaluation Ranking Board. Not going to lie, that stung. It felt like I was right back in Sasebo, and the feeling was not a good one.

HM2 Nick Slagel had a baby girl, Elizabeth Jane, and she's healthy.

Postscript: This was a post that told me a lot of where I was in my mind. I was torn between wanting to relax where I could and keep pushing. I chose the latter because we are taught from a young age to play until you hear the whistle. Thinking of it another way, I remember the Mel Gibson movie We Were Soldiers *(2002) and watching the leader be the first one on the field of battle and last one off. I had not yet left the arena, and therefore my hat was still there. Leaving Qatar to go back to Japan would have saved so much time and was so logical, but as we will see, COVID would strike again.*

FITZ

There are many things I enjoy that may seem mildly odd to the next person. For example, how ink from an expensive pen soaks into the paper or the smell of a library are things I found that not many people notice let alone enjoy. It's these little oddities about ourselves I find so interesting in people if we only take the time to get to know them. Then there are the elements to life that we can universally get behind, but on the surface level can't seem to figure out why. This is when I want to think about not only the movies, but stories in general. Why do we like them, and how have some stood the test of time?

With enough YouTube essays, I have come to learn that there are particular mechanics involved that make a story good and make us care about them. Within these pages, we have come across many characters in my story, and because of the nature of it being a transcribed copy of a diary, there is not nearly enough character development. What we do not get to see is the growth and journey I had with most of these characters. Only they are not characters, they are real people who had people back home who missed and loved them as I had my own. It's because of their humanity that I had the choice on how to feel about them. It's because of my humanity that I did not always do right by them or perform due diligence in assessing who they really were, let alone write about it for others to see.

Lieutenant Commander Kathleen Fitzgerald, Nurse Corps, United States Navy Reserves, was the epitome of these shortcomings. Easily, without question, she received the most unfair treatment of my pen, and the most haunting part for me is we never saw the development of our journey. There were some things in my journal that I left on the editing room floor because they ignored the fact that someone else was on the other side of what I had to say. One of my favorite parts when I look back at a particular duty station is noticing the arcs of my journey with the people I worked with. If I had to submit a David Letterman "Top Ten" list of things I was most proud of during my time with

Whiskey Rotation, my own character arc with LCDR Fitzgerald is among the very top.

Like many problems in our own lives, the person who gets in the way most is ourselves. I am no different, and a lot of it had to do with my helium-inflated ego. When I was not selected as the Public Affairs Officer, "Fitz" had the unfair experience of being under my microscope of ridicule and criticism. I lived in the Land of Make Believe to think that such a role would be given to an enlisted Sailor when an officer also applied for the position. Simply, that isn't how the Navy works, but again, ego. There is a book by Charles Krauthammer, *Things That Matter* (2013), I really enjoy and often think about. How do we as people decide what matters? For 99% of the Whiskey staff, the Public Affairs program didn't matter, but I was hellbent on making it that way. It was my destiny to give Whiskey Rotation a voice and in my head that voice sounded a lot like my own and no one else's, and again, ego.

It takes reflection and concentration, but I have learned that I really do enjoy being "The Guy." This is probably why I haven't run for a committee seat or office of anything besides president. What my time in Whiskey, and journey with Fitz, helped me learn was how to be "the guy who The Guy depends on." For every Steve Jobs, there is a Steve Wozniak. With every "up and out" mentality, there needs to be a "down and in" mind to make the team whole. When the importance of this and the essential nature of teamwork instead of in-house fighting (mostly with me, myself and I) finally clicked in my head, productivity increased, morale rose, and burdens became pleasures. I can be of as much use and importance by being there for support and offering recommendations. Afterall, there is an Oscar specifically for the best supporting actor. When I found peace with being comfortable giving the best recommendation and effort I could to support the PAO, it didn't matter what the outcome was because I performed my role on the team. Some things Fitz agreed with, and other things she wanted to go another direction, but by the end of our time I was able to sleep soundly at night.

To her credit, Fitz was nothing but kind to me. Although confirmed only through third party sources, she even nominated me for an award. Of course, she had her way of going about business that, for lack of a better word, was annoying. Who doesn't have their quirks though? They are the spices to relationships that make life interesting. I know for a fact that I am not always a peach to work with, nor am I the most fun to be around. My kids still think I'm a god, my wife still loves me, and although I'm third in line behind the former two in my parents' eyes, they still like me too. Fitz is no different, she was not some statistical anomaly that needed to be published in some peer-reviewed journal. Everyone in Whiskey was thrown together and wished the best of luck and expected to be professionals. In the case of Fitz and I, it took a little longer, but we made it work.

Lastly, there is a saying I like that really helped me get to the other side of the deployment, and that's "a high tide raises all ships." When times are good, and everyone is able to benefit, the entire team benefits. Because we were able to find a point of equilibrium, Fitz and I, the entire command was able to see our best work come out. I was much more word-driven for *The Whiskey Ration* newsletter, and she liked pictured content more. It was her suggestion that I could start another publication if I wanted to see more articles, and that is how *The Thirsty Camel* was conceived. On the other hand, we were never short on word count or article ideas.

Issue # 10

DEFINITELY NOT A NATO ROLE 3 MMU PUBLICATION

RELEASED THE SAME DAY THE MORALE GREW LEGS AND LEFT

Special points of interest:

- Sean in MEDLOG changed his shampoo to Pert in order to add that extra bounce.
- HM1 Wilson is 42 years old today. Wish him well.
- I like half of you half as much as you'd like, and like less than half of you half half as much as you deserve.

Inside this issue:

Anchor Math	2
Hague Announcement	2
Space Cadet	2
Story about Nutty	3
Supernatural Sightings	3
Dodgeball Name	3
Long Laundry Tale	4

THE THIRSTY CAMEL

EVERYONE WANTS TO BE A HILLBILLY, UNTIL ITS TIME TO DO HILLBILLY SHIT

Not all heroes wear capes. The same sentiment can be said for the hillbillies of the world, especially those who inhabit within the Whiskey Rotation.

Our very own Morale, Welfare and Recreation Committee sponsored a bonfire of things to try and lift the spirits of the homesick crew. This was their first mistake.

With a horseshoe of favorite long cut chaw, the only HM3 James Writer did the only thing he was bred to do.

Before the Thirsty Camel dives into the specifics of the story, it is important to establish context to HM3's story. With no better phrasing at hand of the English language, he is a straight up hick.

Although there are many breeds of this subculture of humans, he is of the Maryland variety although there is a common tongue spoken between the different species which roam the United States.

During the peaceful bonfire where

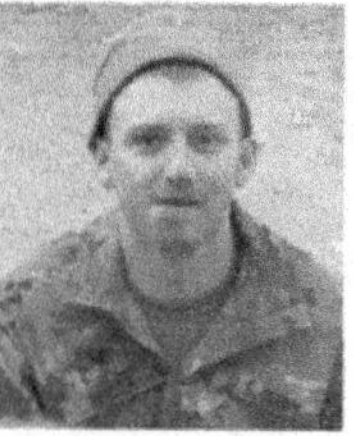

the wanting staff assembled to relax and enjoy the moment, Petty Officer Writer took it upon himself to do what hillbillies do, and look for shit to blow up.

It did not take long before the plan to throw an oxygen tank into the flames became not only the most appealing, but singular thought which ran through his mind.

From the crowd another hillbilly was heard to say that they observe Earth Day by burning tires back on the farm.

Everyone wants to be a hillbilly, as if it is a badge of honor. Where it takes obvious courage to do the stupid stunts they believe are funny, hillbillies are cautionary tales to the rest of the literate world.

Still, to have the sack they do leads to just one conclusion, and that is that everyone wants to be a hillbilly until it's time to do hillbilly shit.

DON'T HAVE TO LEAVE, BUT CAN'T STAY HERE

As the Whiskey Rotation starts its descent from cruising altitude and marches its way toward the landing pattern, there are many mixed feelings at the Thirsty Camel offices.

That is why we feel it best to buzz the tower just one more time, so to speak.

After Issue 10, there will be just one more release of the best news in all of Kandahar. The writers are saddling up for a real doozy, and will strive to perform at the same level as all of its preceding issues. Something about sustained superior performance.

What can be disclosed is that it will be the same length as every other issue, but there will a slight twist to the format.

It's closing time, like every other shop around this base. It's time to move on. The Thirsty Camel says it's closing time. You do not have to go home, but you can't stay here.

Much thanks to the ridiculously long leash which has been extended in order to bring a few laughs when nothing about our deployment was funny. It has been a sincere pleasure to produce this sort of content and share it.

The way the Camel brought so much joy has exceeded every expectation this experiment has started out envisioning. It has been one of the most gratifying poorly managed expectations a three hump chump could have ever asked for. Thank You.

THE THIRSTY CAMEL

Page 2

"A Beautiful Mind"

Some nobody, just another jerk-off Harvard loser.

CHIEF AT APPLIES FOR HARVARD MATH PROGRAM

Anchors don't sink under pressure. They rise to the occasion.

Chief Melvin Atangan has made the bold decision to consider applying to the Harvard Math Program after successfully completing the pharmacy's past Controlled Substance Inventory Board, or CSIB for those in the "biz."

"Normally this stuff is really easy," the Senior Enlisted Leader allegedly said, "it's so easy that COT could have done it, but you know what rolls downhill."

It's true, Chief AT is the most junior ranking member to be eligible to count all the narcotics, but The Camel digresses on that small factoid.

A perfect day for CSIB normally consists of four solid hours of simple addition and subtraction. To be fair, the first hour is drinking coffee and Sailorization with the pharmacy techs. The next hour is waiting for LCDR Deguzman to finish his cage fighting exercises from the comfort of his own room.

This was no normal day however. There were paradoxes that would have made Sir Isaac Newton cringe and John, not Jed, Nash roll over in his grave.

Good thing the Good Chief was at the ready though and put all those squats to good use because he placed the CSIB board on his back and carried the day.

Being at the bottom of the CSIB hierarchy, he was expected to do all the summing and deducting, and like a neurosurgeon without kidney stones, stood his ground, and a local legend was created.

"The pharmacy is my war zone, and its walls make up my Roman Coliseum," snarked Chief.

"LCDR Kathleen Fitzgerald should indeed be let out of the dog house for her actions"

THE HAGUE MAKES BIG ANNOUNCEMENT

In a live stream telecast from the Netherlands evening last, the long awaited verdict was announced that LCDR Kathleen Fitzgerald should indeed be let out of the dog house for her actions in connection with the way she has coercively gotten so many people to buy t-shirts.

The one shirt that says, "Senior promised me a sweet award, but all I got was this shirt instead," is by far the best selling item among the enlisted ranks.

There was wide speculation that the Public Affairs Officer was threatening to have CAPT Klinger write an article about them if they would not donate to the "Cruise Book Fund." Believing that a corpse could knock out a better draft than Whiskey's 'deuce,' a large sum has been contributed to the initiative.

What was also discussed was of course the running joke that PAO left her gun outside, but according to the International Court of Justice, "That shit isn't funny no more, cut it out and find new material to satire."

More to the point, from this day forth to the last, not another mention will be made of that reminder of humanity.

We are all excited to get a copy because it means this shit show will be over.

Some space cadet hanging onto the moon

Everyone is a genius. But if you judge a fish by its ability to climb a tree, it will live its whole life believing that it is stupid

SPACE CADET ARBOLEDA

If you see the Emergency Department's very own HM2 Arboleda, extend for a firm handshake because he is the going to great places.

It has been rumored by multiple sources that he has submitted his transfer paperwork to leave the DON and link up with the newest Department of Defense, the Space Force.

"I think it's time I send my talents elsewhere," said the salty Second Class.

No one was more sad to hear the news than Arbie's very own sea daddy HM2 Rodriguez. According to sources close to Rod, there was a long discussion about the jump from the world's greatest Navy to the world's biggest joke.

"Look," said the last man in Afghanistan to discover a hair clippers, "if you stick with it, this time next year you'll be putting on anchors."

On the opposite side of the spectrum, no one danced later into the night than PS2 Krombach who had to do the paperwork.

"I have been so busy with this bullshit I haven't had time to shave!!!!" "!!!!!!!!!!!!!!!!!!!!!!!!!!!!!!!!!!!!!!" the thankful Pay Officer shyly admitted in an email to the Thirsty Camel.

Whether you sink or swim, float in zero gravity or pack sand, we could all reach for the stars like HM2, and may there be mercy granted for his future endeavors. At least that's how The Camel heard it!

PME INITIATES INTERPLANETARY PATIENT TRANSPORT

The Thirsty Camel has never been secretive about its admiration for the transportation talents of our PME Champions, LCDR Paula Easton and LT Lori Quinn. But now, The Camel has learned through a deep-state, cloistered, and buttoned -down-real-tight secret source that the MARS 2020 Rover Mission included a brave patient volunteer whom our exemplary PME spirited onto the manifest.

The patient, a COVID positive squirrel who had tired quickly of reading 10 year old Guideposts and consuming red licorice in USO isolation, jumped at the opportunity to break loose.

"I'm one of those guys who can't sit still for more than a few minutes," he proudly asserted. "Even if I got free tickets to Hamilton, I wouldn't go!"

LCDR Easton and LT Quinn, feeling sorry for their clandestine friend, used a little known TPMC/PECC/ACLS/TC2GUI/WhatsApp/NIH loophole to include him on the July 30th Cape Canaveral lift-off as a COVID treatment research project.

The stowaway agreed to report his temp and oxygen saturations daily and to immediately let NASA know if he loses his sense of smell.

Easton & Quinn certified him to drive the Mars Rover by observing him peel donuts with the PME van in the Cambridge DFAC parking lot and he was off.

Our unnamed and nonexistent source, expressed his admiration for the 2 Whiskey Nurses, stating, 'Those 2 can work miracles!', then quickly denied he said anything.

Congratulations to our 'stellar' PME!

Squirrel in a space suit. Was rather hard finding this pic to pair with the article.

Nutty the COVID-positive squirrel in uniform prior to launch

SIGHTINGS OF JOHN PAUL JONES REVEALED

To be a government agency two things much happen. The first is that you cannot be efficient, logical, or without a mountain of bureaucracy. The second, and this is the most important, is it must be with secrets.

The Department of the Navy has tried its damnest to keep their secret of supernatural sightings among the Role 3 deckplates just that.

Luckily The Thirsty Camel is the tip of the spear in uncovering the truth.

After a late night bender of Near Beers, LCDR Warner swears on his children's lives that he saw the ghost of John Paul Jones working on his short game with the golf clubs which line his office.

"Tom," the Captain allegedly said, "this office is packed with so much shit that I am pretending it's a miniature golf course."

Although that part of the article is an absolute joke, LCDR Warner is never in Role 3 after 1430 on any given day, on a quiet night if one were to listen carefully, the words of the past come to life.

"Role 3 turns into a night at the museum," said one tech who actually works a full day's work, "the walls may be bare, but they bleed some really profound memories." Cherish this time we had, Whiskey.

"Role 3 turns into a night at the museum… the walls may be bare, but they bleed some really profound memories."

ICU NAMES DODGEBALL TEAM NAME

Earlier this week, the Intensive Care Unit hosted a ceremony to officially announce its team name for the KAF Dodgeball Tournament.

Team Co-Captain LCDR Claudine Bansil was ecstatic for the event for two reasons. One, there would be lots of food. Two, there would be lots of people to feed.

"I sort of feel whole again by whipping up a meal cooked with love," said the ICU nurse.

For the KAF wide tournament, the ICU team will be named the Viper Pit.

"It's biting," said a sarcastic LT Scott Byrd.

Being able to play in a dodgeball tournament is a miracle in itself, but the base brass was dedicated to roll out its team name too in conjunction with the ICU's ceremony.

Team TAAC-South will be called the "Stone Hearts."

"It's not a joke, said the base PAO." We were going to host an ice-hockey tournament and call ourselves the Ice Kings, but decided that dodgeball was more within our budget. "It's logic."

Viper Pit coach HM1 Blades is calling for a pitchers and catchers meeting tomorrow at 1500 in the ICW.

"We're looking gooodd," giggled the first year coach, and KAF vet.

Dodgeball villain here.

The ICU. "WE'RE BETTER THAN YOU, AND WE KNOW IT!"

Whiskey Helps.

THE OKTOBERFEST THAT COULD HAVE BEEN?

Please take a moment to imagine a world that included our stop to Germany, in October of all months, after nothing less than a stressful deployment.

Queue the John Lennon because The Camel is imagining the cigar smoke, the hugs, the real beer and the passing around our favorite memes.

Imagine the cool days and chill nights, sitting around fires and carrying our steins as if they were our first born. Take a moment to breathe in the German air, the laughter, the relief and the thought we no longer have to wear a gun on our hips.

Imagine LT Veatch playing "Never Have I Ever" and CDR Self nursing four fingers of brandy or whatever the Hell Okies drink. Imagine LCDR Van Pelt being a nice guy and everyone walking around believing that in a short couple of days they will be home to warm embraces of their families and loved ones.

Now snap your fingers and wake up. You're going to a hotel room in Norfolk. F@ck COVID and the horse it rode in on.

LUCKY STRIKE TO SPONSOR EOT AWARDS

It has been decided that after a careful survey of the best sponsors to host the End of Tour Ceremony, that Lucky Strike Cigarettes would be selected. No one is happy with this decision, especially the lab techs because they like to smoke those candy-ass cigarettes.

The End of Tour Awards is a traditional ceremony held by all departing Role III rotations. Last year's sponsor was the Department of the Army's Daughters of the Bronze Star Committee, a private non-profit that has insider tracks to the highest levels of Army leadership.

"What could be better than a firm handshake and a soft pack of Lucky's?," promoted Senior Chief Wink.

Clearly anything would be better, an EOT colonoscopy by Dr. Prakash would be more enlightening than this, but like so many other facets of this deployment, we have to carry on smartly and play the hand we're dealt. We're Whiskey, Trojans of Tabata or whatever the Hell those lunatics subscribe to calling themselves.

THE CASE OF THE MISSING LAUNDRY

Promotional Poster for "The Wire" because it's an awesome show and I wanted to show some homage.

Command duty is typically a straight-forward endeavor albeit a time consuming perspiration inducing task that we all share in.

The situation became a bit dicey for Team Teruya/Self a couple of days ago.

Upon checking in the dirty laundry to the industrial house of washing, it was eventually determined that there was one bag short of the official check-in muster.

After searching as high and low as their feeble bodies would allow inside the van, CDR Self had the bright idea to search the top of the van because according to him, the vans don't drive fast enough for anything to fly off. He has apparently saved more than one Near Beer in this fashion.

Despite their valiant efforts to seeing the mission accomplished, it was quickly crystal clear that the missing bag, belong to Arkansas' favorite son LT Byrd, was AWOL.

In the face of a total FUBAR situation, the Provost Marshal's Office was contacted and a BOLO (Be On the Look Out) dispatch was radioed to all mobile units.

As the dragnet was underway, and flights were recalled back to base in the case of an international heist for the good lieutenant's underwear, LT Byrd was finally questioned regarding the errant duffle.

With a slight application of professional pressure to the persecution, the Byrd-man may have suggested that it was plausible he had in fact logged in the laundry onto the muster log, but was too absent-minded or considerate enough to the duty crew to actually put the bag in question into the large white bin.

Holding the Department Head accountable for his actions, the incident has been passed up the chain of command.

Senior Chief can't believe another Junior Officer's bullshit is back on his desk, the Executive Officer laughed it off because that's what he does best, and the CO, well, we don't talk about what the CO does or does not do within these pages.

15 Aug 2020
Day 180

Two more days until Rastall Boy #3 enters the world. I've gone to lengths to tell Saori that she will be picking the name when the baby comes. I've given my favorites, so hopefully she will pick one of them. Either way, it will ultimately be her choice.

Finally got around to watching *The Green Book* (2018) last night. It was well-acted, although predictable.

Starting to really put on the press for packing my things to be mailed. The post office closes in two weeks. Everything is closing.

We had our group photo today for the cruise book. HM1 LaPenna was not present. He said he overslept. Then the hospital had a mass casualty drill. HM1 LaPenna did not attend this either. I feel like I'm in an awkward place because I notice him acting weird lately, but I'm his subordinate. Not like he was suicidal, but off his game. Today's couple of mishaps only proved my point. Rank has its privileges though, because I would have been turned inside out if that was ever me. Maybe he will be too in some room I'm not a part of, but I'm concerned for him and wish I knew what to do.

The book HM1 Wilson loaned me is done. *Stillness is the Key* might have been the best book on the deployment yet. I'll probably add it to my Christmas gift list for Sailors.

My parents are buying a gun. Makes me glad I live in Japan.

Postscript: Everything is closing. This is charming to recall because most of it was closed. When I talk to Sailors who served on earlier rotations at the Role III, they inevitably ask me if I checked this or that out. It's always a resounding "no." HM1 LaPenna missing that photo shoot was weird, and I ended up talking with him about it. He only showed that he was human, and, like so many of us spread out across the months, found himself in a rut. Allowances were given, to me he had earned it, but it was hot out there and all I wanted was for him to share our misery.

16 Aug 2020
Day 181

This is it. My final night with only two sons. By this time tomorrow I will be talking about son #3. It's a delirious feeling, hard to catch on paper, but it goes back, I think, ultimately to Saori, and not only my love for her, but admiration for her too. Her will, grit, and drive help make me a better man every day, and how she continues to carry our family, especially while we are apart. Makes me cherish her even more.

Last night I watched *The Greatest Showman* (2017) starring Hugh Jackman. Today I bought its soundtrack. Not sure what it is about musicals, but they always get me in the feels. The last three I saw, *La La Land* (2016), *Les Misérables* (2012), and now this one, always get my allergies flaring up. I awarded it a 9/10 on IMDB.com.

Also talked to an old friend, Kelcey Heath. She's divorcing her husband, who I know too, and we talked about it. What else could I do except share some YouTube videos to help convey what I wanted to say. She said those videos helped a lot, both of them, and that felt good.

Mailed three packages home. Two of them I paid for priority postage. Almost all my "extra" stuff is now gone with one more box to go. This is perfect timing because the new rumor is the CENTCOM four-star general wants to keep the hospital open as a Role III. More to follow.

Capped off my day out of bed with a lively and robust video chat with Dr. Solomon.

Postscript: The Greatest Showman *is a soundtrack I still listen to and love every song. It's just long enough for a good spin on the treadmill. More importantly it is a film that has inspired me to do more, which we will see in later pages. There is nothing easy or convenient about being married to my wife. It does not take away that she is the best thing that has ever happened to me. She is the most loving wife and the best mother. When speaking about fidelity with junior Sailors, I often cite that a good wife "loves you when you weren't very lovable and didn't leave you when she had every opportunity and reason to." That is my wife in one sentence. Rumors during this time were crazy, and it soon became simply entertaining more than anything.*

THE THIRSTY CAMEL

Ah yes, the pride and joy of the deployment. It was also the dark horse morale booster I had no idea was needed. My old friend Rich once told me that some of the things he says is purely for his own entertainment. *The Camel* started out as that, a medium for me to entertain myself. It obviously grew to something much more than it was originally intended to be, and in a way its success gave me license to draft this book.

It's interesting to me because I never really considered myself funny. I'm not even the funniest person in my family, my brother Dylan is given that honor. Why then would I ever attempt to write a satirical newsletter? There were a couple of sources of inspiration along the way. *The Onion* is given the most obvious credit. My high school history teacher, Steve Argo, had an "*Onion's* greatest hits" collection in his room, and between lectures in the downtime of the class I'd flip through its pages, always being impressed at the creativity involved to develop such zany and clever stories.

Again, by no means am I a witty person, but I soak up witticisms like a sponge and always try to store them like a bank to be used later. These little nuggets of rhetorical gold often come out in mentorship moments or when developing an argument. Sometimes they work, and other times it would have been best to keep my mouth shut, but either way you'll never score on the shot you never take. That's a philosophy, keep at-bat appearances high and keep swinging, eventually something will connect. With practice and study, anyone would be amazed by how many hits they can get. There are too many people to specifically credit, but it's a case study of how people's words matter, and someone is always listening.

Things started to become bolder when I took over as the Public Affairs Officer for the clinic in Sasebo. Everyone talked about a newsletter, but I had never seen one that was sustained for a period of time. Because I was trying to break the mold, become innovative and be different, I decided to add a newsletter onto Sasebo's Public Affairs program. It would run in-house and be published at the beginning of each month. Commanders and leaders love newsletters, and I felt there was enough content on a monthly basis to create a sustainable product. Because we published on the first of the month, we would be rolling out our "April Fools" issue, which was going to be completely satire. The Role III deployment railroaded these plans, and I was left without a platform yet full of ideas.

Next was joining the Public Affairs Office for the deployment. I knew I wanted to write. What I didn't know about myself was I didn't play well with others (see the "Fitz" chapter). Because of LCDR Fitzgerald's recommendation to start my own publication, I was back on track, and the steam kept building. It started with all the downtime we had in Texas. As a huge fan of people-watching at airports and other public venues, I began to make little stories in my head of everyone on the deployment based primarily on their displayed behaviors. Some stories were boring, and they'd be immediately trashed, but others piqued my interest, and I went as far down the rabbit hole as I could until there was something worth jotting down to remember for a later time.

At the airport terminal in Qatar on the way into Afghanistan, I had my favorite headlines on a scratch piece of paper. Like any good journalist, I had to triangulate my material to make sure it was credible. My mind and ego had already signed off on the project, so I brought in HM3 James Writer. He liked the idea. Initially, I thought it was going to be more of a partnership, but not everything falls where you might think it will. I was so full of ideas and wanted to be creative, so I did not end up using another writer until the final couple of issues. Turns out other people like to be creative such as Commander John Mayberry, Commander Phil Self, and Lieutenant Scott Byrd.

As touched on in the journal, I honestly thought my first issue would be my last. Commander Judd Nash mentioned something about a similar type of periodical on another deployment of his called *The Sandy Goat.* Originally, I wanted to use that title as a tip of the hat to the rotations before Whiskey, but I couldn't remember the title. That is how *The Thirsty Camel* got its name. Since it was a stand-alone publication in no way tied to official media, I always added the subtext: DEFINITELY NOT A ROLE III MMU PUBLICATION. It was the sea lawyer in me coming out and protecting myself, but the subtext stuck and made its way into this book title too.

History will come to show that *The Camel* became wildly popular. It spoke to many people. I made fun of the obvious things that not many people could bring up. By building this persona, I was able to explore the problems, triumphs, and failures in a light-hearted way. Imagine sitting in church and the old lady in the pew across from you farts. Saying the HAZMAT team was brought in would make fun of a light subject, while in a normal world nothing would have been said at all, out loud.

The end to *The Camel* was almost a badge of honor. After 10 issues it had gotten farther than I ever would have dreamed. I had people asking me to send them electronic copies. I saw people clip out stories about them over their desks. Friends in the military gave it high praise even though they did not know any of the backstories that I thought made the article funny to begin with. When I was told that I couldn't write *The Thirsty Camel* on government computers because I should be working on work when I was at work, I had no idea how high that order came from, and frankly I didn't care. I had made my mark on the deployment, and if there was one thing I can be remembered by, it's that newsletter.

18 Aug 2020
Day 182 & 183

Well, isn't this all fine and dandy today. Of all the days to miss an entry, yesterday was not supposed to be one of them. To be honest, I felt a little weird to write about a child with no name. We solved that problem by welcoming Oliver Gregory Rastall into the family. The Japanese middle name is still being hashed out, but the English names are submitted.

For the historical record, the final four names were Francis, Levi, Theodore and Oliver. From my 42-name bracket I created in Qatar back in May, Oliver was the 10th seed. I think what I like most about his name is his nickname, Ollie. There is no one who he is named after like how Levi was going to be for HM1 Levi Arcaira. As much as I liked Theodore, anyone who knows me would think even that was a little much, even for a guy who loves TR (that would have been his initials too) as much as I do. Plus, the joke is I had a girlfriend in high school who left me for a guy named Theo, and I wouldn't be able to nickname him that. Francis was after Francis Underwood who is a horrible man, but a great character. Plus, I don't know if my son would ever be Pope so there's that. The only connection I have to Oliver is my grandfather's tractor that he called Ollie. It is hardly cause to name a son Oliver except for the high regard he had in Ollie to get the job done. I thoroughly like Oliver, but also totally can sign off on Ollie too.

I suppose there is Ollie North, but I just found out about him today after the fact. Also, I have never read *Oliver Twist*, yet.

Saori is doing well. She is sore as expected, but she sent a picture of her ability to nurse. I think with mothers that is a big deal and a huge accomplishment. Because of the COVID restrictions at the hospital, they are not allowing any visitors, and that is a bummer. I haven't seen the big brothers since Saori was admitted, but she sent screenshots of the boys looking at him. Atticus appears the most curious, and Josiah looks like he is saddling up for extra big brother duties.

Haven't called Wisco yet. Mail Call yesterday too. Big day. A very thoughtfully crafted box by my friend Kallie Lane who I learned was the mystery postcard writer. Then there is a care package from my mom and dad. Christina Solomon penned a thoughtful letter as she always has before, but then there was the grand finale of my littlest cousin Emilia who sent a letter. It was my first from all the cousins of that era.

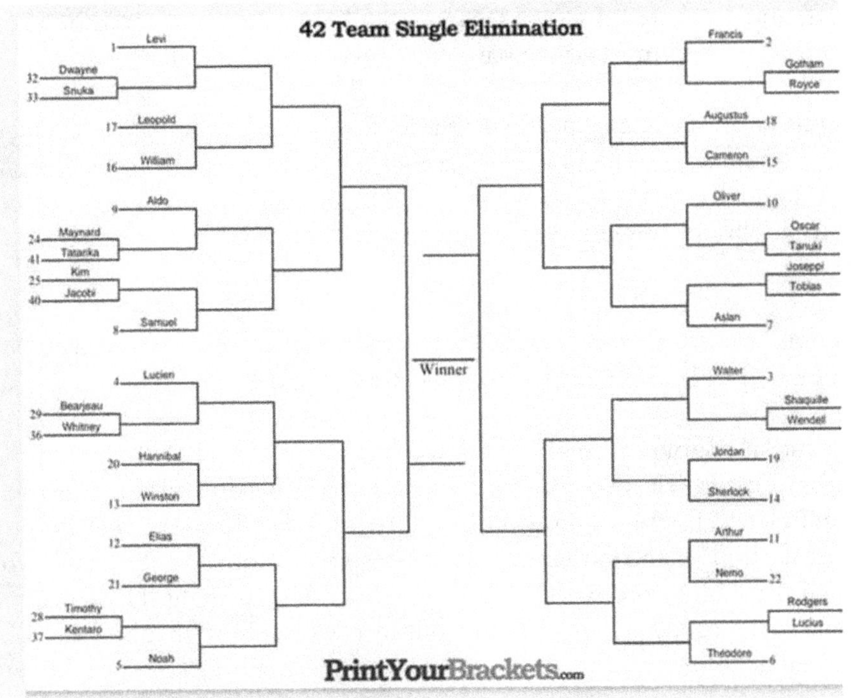

Postscript: I often wondered how parents could have a baby and not have the name on standby. Well, it happened to us. I called Saori and was like, "What's the name?!" She was like, "I don't know yet." This was crazy to me, but we eventually got it sorted out. I was not special to have a baby on deployment. I believe there were five new fathers in Whiskey Rotation. Some were first timers, and a couple were seasoned veterans such as myself. Some were able to leave early to ensure they didn't miss the birth, and some like me had to endure the full deployment treatment. I'm happy for the those who were able to leave early; being present for the birth of a child is an angelic moment.

19 Aug 2020
Day 184

This day turned from boring to interesting really, really fast. It all started with not being able to sleep last night. As I lay in bed my 0400 alarm went off, and I debated if I could stay awake long enough to catch breakfast and then sleep most of the day. Well, I woke up at 1130.

Quickly manscaped one final time before packing my clippers. Maybe two boxes to go. Then I had a very nice talk with Saori. Ollie was sleeping next to her, and we did a lot of talking about my life after I return. Hopefully, I'll be able to live up to these expectations when that day comes.

Found out some really good news. September 12, twenty-four days, and a max of eight more duty nights, we are flying out.

Wrote a couple of emails. First was to Master Chief Branch. I shared what I could tell about the movement, Oliver's birth, and what I've been up to lately, but saved most of the last part for *The Whiskey Ration* to speak for itself. The second email was the response from Master Chief Greg Fall. I told his wife Apryl about the namesake last night. His email was endearing as always. It's hard to put into words how thankful I am for some people.

Today I threw out my back. Spasms are crazy, but I've been down this road before. The second to last thing about my day was an emergency recall to the hospital. Was on the phone with Big Dan, always great talking to him. Gunshot wound, non-American. He'll live. Doing laundry now.

Postscript: It is hard to imagine what deployment life was like before the internet. It makes the world so much smaller. Part of me wished I could have experienced the full treatment, but parts of me are thankful too. I am proud of the namesakes for all of my children; there are few higher nods of respect than to name a child after someone. Greg Fall is no different, and so much of what I have has been because he has been in my life. Every sinner has a future, and every angel has a past is the way I look at it.

20 Aug 2020
Day 185

Today was a duty day, and yet it was for the most part a restless one. Technically we have two patients admitted, but the level of involvement from the pharmacy is actually minimal.

The guy who was shot four times is using MiraLAX for the only scheduled medication and that is a ward stock item. After whipping up an Ancef (antibiotic) to batch and one dilaudid bag, that was it. HM1 LaPenna was in good spirits today, and that was fun to see.

My roommate on the other hand, not so much. I heard what the source of this trouble might be, but for the sake of dignity I won't repeat it here. It does however pain me when I see someone, especially who I live with, working through some adversity.

LT Kevin Veatch sent a PayPal gift for Ollie, and I just looked at the deposit today. It was for $200. Holy smokes. I immediately wrote him a short letter of appreciation. It was the least I could do.

HM1 Wilson was in a spunky mood today. He kept riding me about advancement studying, and when I placed some flags in our quarterdeck in the correct order of precedence, he undid it. I wonder what he was thinking. At first, I was mad, but then curious about what was going through his mind. Was there a lesson to be taught? What was I not seeing? Unfortunately, my confrontation skills leave more to be desired, and I think he's quicker to be defensive.

Postscript: Looking back on this with the benefit of hindsight, I can see how stupid my thinking was. I was literally looking for a problem and found it by getting a reaction so worthy I mentioned it to my diary. I couldn't even prove it was Wilson to begin with, but I had prided myself on my ability to put clues together based on observations. The advancement test in the Navy is a twice-annual exam consisting of 175 questions based on knowledge from our rate and what we should know at the next higher paygrade. Just because you ace the test does not mean you advance because that is only one factor in the process. Things like evaluations (based on a point system), college education, personal awards, and time in rate are entered into a formula. With a high enough score and above the quota set by the Bureau of Navy Personnel each cycle, you advance. Everyone knew I was long in the tooth when it came to my time as a Second Class Petty Officer, and I don't blame Wilson for "encouraging" me.

21 Aug 2020
Day 186

Today is a date I feel I ought to remember for its significance, but I can't seem to place my finger on it. Oh well, pretty easy day.

I woke up at 0745, prepped everything for turnover, and HM1 Wilson cut me loose before I poured my first cup of coffee. Because I made my own special blend of espresso and coffee, I stuck around for one cup. Truth be told, even that was a little hard. There was nothing to do that wouldn't be frowned at work like reading my book or writing *The Thirsty Camel.* Before going home, I mailed the rest of the office things I had in the pharmacy. Just a bunch of coffee and leftovers from care packages that weren't already donated to the communal bowl outside the pharmacy window.

Came home and took a nap pretty fast. Woke up at 1400, went to lunch, got on YouTube for a bit, and then went back to the post office for my next-to-last big box of things. Although I thought it would be my last, it turns out I have room and enough things for one more. I might just take the water heater thingy too.

Even though it is Friday, and therefore steak day at the chow hall, I missed dinner. Just wasn't hungry. At 2000 we had a farewell for CDR Prakash. I knew him, and we were friendly but not close.

Watched *Reservoir Dogs* (1992) for the first-time last night and Brie Larson's Oscar performance in *Room* (2015) tonight.

Postscript: There are a couple of places I abnormally enjoy. It can be traced back to who this book is dedicated to, my mother's mom, Grandma Mongin. She enjoyed the library and the post office. There is a third habit I picked up from her and that's to not mind walking directly into the bank as opposed to using the drive-thru window. In many places I have stated that if I were ever to become "Oprah rich" I would place my philanthropic money in the library systems of America. To me, the post office is such a cool place because of all the services they provide and their ability to get a single letter across the world in less than a week. I just find that amazing.

22 Aug 2020
Day 187

Wow, three naps in one day. That's what I was able to experience today on my day off. If I was ever asked, I know I would say I'm practicing for napping with Ollie. No way Saori would ever let that fly, but a Papa can dream.

I'm listening to *The Greatest Showman* soundtrack, again. I'm borderline obsessed, but I think it is getting some creative juices flowing. "I lie awake in bed, a million ideas dancing in my head" is really speaking to me. I feel responsible to do something with my ideas and somehow share them. Although I messed up the actual lyrics just now, a million dreams really are keeping me awake.

That's why I started to dream and build a possible screenplay. It's about a unit of ragtag reservists trying to work together at a combat hospital. Sounds familiar, doesn't it? Although this journal is the basis for this film, there are definitely parts which need to be glamorized for dramatic effect.

By diverging from a historical piece like this journal, I would be more comfortable with taking creative license. Who knows what will come of it? Probably leave it on top of my pile of never finished projects.

Watched the Denzel movie *Man on Fire* (2004). I did not like the way it was directed. I guess I appreciate cameras that can stand still.

Postscript: One of the selling points to have a third baby was the thought of nap time. I love naps, and yes, Saori hates it when I sneak away for a couple hours every weekend afternoon. She wanted our third child to be a daughter so bad, and I was personally fine with our two healthy boys, but the thought of extending an excuse to take naps for another four to five years meant a lot to me too. I was never going to have more "free time" than I did on that deployment, and I wanted to capitalize on it. Much of what I stress to more junior Sailors is to seize the time they have now when they are unaccompanied (single) without a care in the world except for themselves. Youth is wasted on the young however, and those fleeting moments of opportunity are often noticed only after the time has passed us by.

23 Aug 2020
Day 188

Well, today was an interesting one. I had some trouble falling asleep last night. After writing the first scene of my screenplay, I went back inside, got on YouTube for a bit, and finally went to sleep between 0130-0230. I wasn't tired.

Then at 0500 I heard a very panicked cry of, "I need some help here! Quick!" I got my shoes on as quickly as I could and dashed out the door. Honestly, I thought someone had hung themselves or I somehow slept through a gunshot. As it turned out, Lieutenant Kevin Veatch, the selfless OR nurse, passed out in the bathroom and HM3 Jonathon Gibford either was there or found him. LT hit the back of his head during the fall and no one, from what I know, could figure out what happened. This has me puzzled. The man is as nice as they come, but he gave me a large cash baby gift, and he paid for a hefty amount on HM2 Nick Slagle's baby registry. On top of that he just gave a pair of Bose headphones away to HM3 Wes Alden. They are apparently valued at $300. Now he's passing out in the bathroom? It seems all very coincidental, and I let HM1 LaPenna know my thoughts.

Besides that, it was essentially dead. I wrote a few more pages in my screenplay and did a training on the pharmacy with the Role I Army kids.

Postscript: When everyone was putting their stories together after the fact about what they experienced during the bathroom incident, I heard the best story of them all. It was HM2 Jesse John who, hearing the cry for help, jumped from his bed, grabbed his sidearm, and ran into the hall in just his underwear. Had the situation been different and there been an actual fire fight, that would have been a story that would be echoed in every bar from every man on the deployment. Unfortunately for Jesse, that was not the case. Kevin Veatch is a reservist, a bachelor all his life, and might love Kentucky more than I love Wisconsin. We've exchanged care packages since the deployment and still keep in touch. With so much going on, it was easy to make the logical leap to assume the worst. He is fine and in good spirits. The difference in Roles depends on the capabilities. We were a Role III, meaning that we had a neurosurgeon and internal medicine doctor plus an ICU large enough to sustain and hold multiple casualties. Role I is a less-capable platform, but we shared the same building.

24 Aug 2020
Day 189

Happy birthday to me. After thirty-three laps around the sun, one might think I had it figured out, but age is just a number. I wish I could have celebrated in any way, but that didn't happen. Instead, I watched the pharmacy for HM1 Wilson until 1900 as the E-6s were at the E-5 Evaluation Ranking Board.

As I was telling myself all day, as long as a favorable ranking comes of this then this will all be funny one day. At the time it was the longest day ever. Nothing I couldn't handle, plus LCDR Deguzman was with me 90% of the day, but it was a long day. I was tired in my mind.

Another patient came in today, an Afghan national. Story is he was at home, the doorbell rang, and one of his kids answered. They went to get him, and he was shot in his home. What the hell? How harrowing is that thought?

Ollie and Saori came home today. Lots of good pictures and videos, and sadly we got into our first argument in a long time. Looking back on it, I realize that I could have been more empathetic and just listened to her tell me her problems. Nope, not me, of course not. I had to fix it and marginalize her dilemma. Although the phone call was abruptly ended by me, I tried to rebound with a thoughtful message.

Postscript: This day was one filled with anxiety. The Whiskey Rotation had more Second Classes than any other rank. All said, there were 20 of us. It was and always is interesting to see a peer group jockeying for a spot. For Navy evaluations, only the top 20% of those evaluated can earn the highest evaluation rating called an "EP," or Early Promote recommendation. Second is "MP," or Must Promote, and the baseline standard is called a "P," for Promotable. Anything below that is a problem. Evaluation recommendations bring more points and a higher the score when it comes to advancement. The overall process for advancement is bit complicated to someone who is not used to it. Probably like any job, the best Sailors are not always the ones who get advanced. It's not what you know, it's what you can prove. I digress; I was stressed this day because in a way everything I was doing was leading up to this judgement at the ranking board.

25 Aug 2020
Day 190

If I thought yesterday was rife with first world problems, then I was mistaken because that was actually today.

It was a day of pettiness on my end looking back on it. So, I promised my sister, Rachael Koontz, to watch her favorite movie, 1993's *The Secret Garden.* As a boy, my family had a VHS copy, and although it goes against my goal of only watching movies I've never seen while here in Afghanistan, a promise was a promise, and I watched it last night. Today I bought the soundtrack, it was that nice and refreshing.

Went to bed late and woke up early for a PAO meeting. One issue left, but for 10 pages. My idea for a superlative page will take up two, and I have to give 20 recommendations so the team will select 12 and we will put out that list for everyone in a popular vote.

Then I mailed an ensign to my Uncle Gordie, but I also mailed arguably my last box. Maybe I'll send more flags too. Then I got a haircut, and we had a mass casualty drill. HM2 Jesse John said I was looking a little pale, and it was because I was mentally beat.

Got home, laid in bed, and turned on my Wi-Fi to see Senior Chief wanted all Second Classes in the hospital for a meeting in 40 minutes. I was mad, but mostly because the meeting took longer waiting for it to happen than anything.

Luckily it was Taco Tuesday for lunch. I called home and took a very solid three-hour nap.

Postscript: There I was being complacent. Off running around doing errands, and the slightest inconvenience set the tone for the entire article. Gordie's mother had passed around the same time I had the flag flown. Instead of mailing it home to my boys, I thought it would be more meaningful if I sent it to him instead. He is an Army veteran and I thought he would appreciate it. Turns out later on he did. That meeting was for a gift to a Chief; I'm not sure why we even had the meeting, but I was just inconvenienced, nothing more.

26 Aug 2020
Day 191

My birthday was only two days ago, but it seems like forever. I felt like time slowed to a crawl, and when I think about how far away September 12 is, it just seems so far away.

We all received our order modifications, and we have a departure date on them, Sept 12. Although I immediately sent the orders encrypted to HMCM Branch, his reply was not very enthusiastic because I don't have an itinerary to Japan yet. So it was a little deflating, but I don't blame him; the orders really told him nothing. They did however tell me one thing, an end date.

Our replacement team is expected to arrive on the 28th of August. Who knows though; I have to prepare for the worst, but hope for the best.

Saori wants to put Josiah into Cub Scouts and I'm all about it. She was able to get Oliver enrolled into military medical today. I guess I just miss them all back at home.

HM1 Wilson is burning some midnight oil working on evals. He thought that I'll be happy with where I was ranked. He then went on to counsel me on a number of things, such as the fitness standard, pissing people off, and the subjectivity of boards. It just seemed there was more talked about on what I could improve on, rather than where I was strongest. Confusing conversation, but sometimes that is life.

Almost there. Taught an Enlisted Advancement Program course on pharmacy too.

Postscript: This was not simply the beginning of the end, this was the end. The wait was over, we now had dates. I missed those conversations with HM1 Wilson and LaPenna. Both offered so much perspective and insight. LCDR Deguzman was the consummate officer too, knowing when to be the O-5, and when to remember he was enlisted once too. Wilson and LaPenna heard me complain so much about everything, they deserved the awards they received at the end. Hopefully I made up for it by my performance, but I was a fat ball of frustrated desperation over the course of this entire deployment.

27 Aug 2020
Day 192

This is turning into a nice little streak of consecutive days putting in an entry. In a way it feels really nice. One piece at a time, or so the man in black says.

There wasn't a whole lot that happened today. At 0130 I was woken up by Role I for an anthrax shot for a Navy Role III nurse! I was exceptionally upset and surprised about who it was because I would have otherwise thought this person would have been more considerate of my time. It was blatant disrespect, one disparity I can't stand between officers and enlisted. No one is saying they can't have the shot, but how about before taps or after reveille. 0130 for an immunization? Unreal.

Then I got to take off from work by 1000. Felt good, but probably felt better because I got to have nothing planned today. No meetings, no obligations, no nothing. It felt joyous. Went home, called Saori and had a good conversation. Then took a solid nap. Woke up to Josiah calling to say goodnight.

My roommate, HM2 Drumheller, came back from duty and let me know there were cheese sticks being served at the galley. He later said he never saw me get out of bed that fast. Overate at dinner and seriously thought about working out, but it's late now.

Watched three HBO documentaries on Olympians mental health, Carrie Fisher, and one about an anorexia clinic.

Postscript: I enjoy learning, and that's why I like documentaries so much. The problem is I also recognize how biased they can be. Cheese sticks were a definite highlight at the chow hall. It pairs up there with Taco Tuesday and Wing Wednesday. One thing I like to say and honestly believe in is if you put in the work, when you do have free time, it'll feel that much better. Today was no different. The bigger point of this entry was the 0130 immunization. Looking back at it, I heavily doubt it was an officer who wished to throw their rank around and not be considerate, but instead was just not aware. They probably read an email for the first time on night shift and immediately walked over to the Role I to receive their shot. Everything else just happened consequently. Why do we fear the worst, or make up the most harrowing stories in our minds before we know all the facts?

THE BRASS

In the Navy, the highest level of leadership is called the "triad," which consists of the Commanding Officer (CO), Executive Officer (XO), and senior enlisted (normally the "Command Master Chief," but in the Whiskey Rotation was the Senior Enlisted Advisor, or "SEA"). In many ways the roles are similar to that of business leadership where the CO is the CEO, the XO is the Senior VP, and the SEA serves as the long-tenured labor union leader who is as salty as they are knowledgeable.

The responsibilities vary between the positions. The Commanding Officer is charged with ultimate authority and final decisions. They can make any decision they feel is best to complete the mission, and generally it has to be a big deal before it can fall on their desk for judgement. For example, because we were in the middle of COVID, it was decided to ban team sports, including basketball. CO's also have bottom line authority on essentially anything that falls under their command but will often delegate authority to a lesser rank while retaining ultimate responsibility.

Executive Officers on the other hand are in many ways the vice principal of commands. They keep the directorate heads aligned with the CO's vision and could be considered a watchdog among the officers in general. In more ways than one, they are being trained by the CO to one day take their own command should they be ambitious enough and have enough years left in their careers. To say they are "groomed" would be a poor choice of words because we are talking about the rank of Captains and Colonels who have established their style, know their road, and foresee much of their own destiny.

Which leaves the Senior Enlisted Advisor to pick up the rest of the top-tier responsibilities. They are charged with establishing good order and discipline throughout the command. No one tells the SEA what to do, and they are often found counseling junior to mid-grade officers on points of improvement. SEA's have a thankless job because they have to gauge the morale of the Sailors in executing the CO's directives. It takes a special person to be light on their feet yet rooted enough by their years of experience to maneuver through their tour.

Ultimately, only crazy people want their jobs. The burden of responsibilities they carry for what they get in return is marginal. They might take the job for a POSSIBLE favorable consideration when promotion boards convene, or an award they'll have to pay extra money to add to their already-towering stack of ribbons on their chests. This is why so much respect is rendered to these three individuals, especially the Commanding Officer. This is also why they seemingly have "the easy life," in the eyes of junior enlisted, or "bluejackets." There is little pause to consider the CO has their lives in their hands and is dealing with much larger issues than having to clean out their own trash can. To me, this is unfortunate because the older I get, the more I get to see how pressed senior leadership is by what is required of them.

I was fortunate to experience a very good triad. Not every Sailor can proudly write that. The three of them together did what was needed to get us to Afghanistan safely and return all together. Because I was able to see my wife and kids again, I have them to thank. The three of them had their own spunky personality and way of conducting the business of Whiskey's day. My normal interaction with the triad was limited, especially the higher up I went on the food chain, and as a result, there were only a few stories which made their way into the journal. These are a couple of those memories.

My Commanding Officer was like any seasoned Sailor, she loved coffee. So much so that we flew a coffee pot from Camp Pendleton, CA, to Fort Bliss, TX, just to be sure she would not be without her beloved cup of morning motivation. While we were in Qatar, everyone was jet lagged to some degree. It helped to want to sleep all day when the sun was highest because it was so hot. Many of us, the Skipper included, would wake up very early and hop over to a spare room we had set up called "the Coffee Mess." Here, the earliest of risers would congregate and share their stories and complaints. When the head honcho came in though, we'd be all smiles and life is great.

She'd sit in a chair and engage in polite conversation, never showing her full hand as a good senior officer should do. I, of course, had other plans. In the Coffee Mess there was a checker/chess/backgammon board left behind by other groups before us. It has always been a serious question of do the Joint Chiefs of Staff ever play the games Battleship or Risk and did the Navy or Army have an advantage? For reasons that are my own, I felt that engaging the Commanding Officer in a game of checkers would somehow settle this question.

To my surprise, she accepted my offer. As an enlisted fellow, I felt the advantage was mine. There was a reason why chess was not offered. As they say, drag them to your level and beat them with experience. It was here between plays that I really got to know my CO. Her past duty stations, critical-thinking process, explanation of the Navy hierarchy, you know, the light conversation topics. The Skipper went along sipping her coffee, pandering to my silly questions, all while beating my ass worse than my daddy ever did.

Never in my life had I been so completely destroyed at checkers. She was pulling moves from nowhere, and there were witnesses to this beatdown. There is no doubt it took a titanic amount of humility to not laugh in my face, but to my luck, the Skipper had what it took. I also realized here the infinite number of other things that had to have been on her mind at the time (when the unit was departing, security, operational stuff) but she not only took the time to play me in a game of checkers but walloped me in the process. That level of thought was very interesting to me and something I will always remember her for. Unfortunately, that was our longest conversation, but for a suspended moment of time, I was able to play my CO in a game of checkers. Only on deployment.

Captain Jeff Klinger was the XO, and he was the anti-XO prototype. We didn't fear him, we loved him. He always had a good story or somehow interjected his personality fittingly into a conversation. In no world would anyone have guessed he was a rank below Admiral if he was seen in civilian clothes. That's just who he was, and he made it work.

CAPT Klinger had this habit of walking; he might have walked the deck plates more than any Whiskey Sailor. He was engaged at the lowest levels. Another habit was pronouncing people's names wrong. I'm Rastall, but it's pronounced more like "Ras-tul." Without fail, he would greet me more along the lines of "RAS-TAAL!!" He would also call the Pay Officer, PS2 Robert Krombach "Krom-batch" (which caught on with other Sailors). He may have respected other people's surnames, but we took it as a term of endearment. You see, on deployment, you have to take the wins where they come.

My best memory, though, of XO was so fast and miniscule, it would take longer to set up the story than explain what happened. I had some troublesome news to share. Although I can't remember what it was, I remember thinking whoever heard it was not going to like the message. I'm horrible at placing my feelings on my forehead, and I'm often ignorant of my own posture when this happens. I literally walked past XO's office door, turned my head to see he was inside as I walked past, and he asked me what the matter was. This was so memorable to me because it showed a) how fast he could read his Sailors and b) was bothered enough to ask. In the chain of command there is a mountain of red tape between me and the XO, but he cared enough to ask. It took me by surprise, and I will forever appreciate the attention to detail. I will always be a Badgers fan, though, no matter how great he thinks UCONN is.

Senior Chief Wink should have his own book written about him, but that is not the Chief way. He ate more crap than anyone else on the deployment. I know in some journal entries he's not written in the best light (to wit, many people got that same shake from me), but as objective as one can be, he was head and shoulders the best pound-for-pound (not inch-for-inch) leader on the deployment. The way he was able to balance the burdens of senior leadership while still being approachable by the most junior Sailor was, to me, nothing short of amazing.

Of the triad, I had the most interaction with Senior Chief Cameron Wink, and that makes sense. His number one priority is the well-being of the enlisted. Specific stories have been mentioned throughout the journal, but there is one observation that was not. Senior had this ability to make you feel better when you are feeling bad. I received this treatment firsthand when I was feeling anxious about promotion and the MAP season. I witnessed it when he was consoling another disappointed Sailor too. He just had this way with words which made you feel better when you needed to hear it most. In another universe he would have made a great chaplain. In other words, he was a good Chief. Maybe not the Chief we deserved, but the one we needed.

29 Aug 2020
Day 193 & 194

The humor is not lost on me that the day after saying something about my consecutive-day streak I go and mess it all up. In my defense that was not the plan, but my roommate, HM2 Drumheller, wanted to try and go to bed early. He is able to sleep best in a dark room, so I told him that I'd wait to hear him snore before I'd turn my lamp back on to journal. As it turns out, I realized I had never seen the Tom Cruise movie *Risky Business* (1983), and by the time it was over it was already 0130. In other words, I was too tired myself! The movie was good, but I think I enjoyed *The Girl Next Door* (2004) more. Probably because I saw it at a more impressionable age, but regardless the two movies have eerily similar plots.

I digress, tonight I want to see *Mission Impossible: Fallout* (2018), but we will see. Lately, I am finding myself with more time on my hands, and that is good. In a way it's relaxing, but on the other hand I'm getting itchy with wanting to be creative. After this I am looking forward to writing a little bit more of the screenplay. Nothing is stopping me from writing letters either I suppose, but I'm not stressed. Well, the bad kind of stress at least.

I walked into work with a lot of good news. For starters, my Lean Six Sigma certification came in an email. Immediately sent my NEC request to the Bureau of Navy Personnel to have it placed into my record.

Then I got an email from my LPO in Sasebo, HM1 Joshua Whicker. He outright offered me the Enlisted Watchbill Coordinator position. After something like six years as the assistant, this has been a dream of mine. Maybe I was given an inch, but I took a mile when I also asked his thoughts about me requesting to be put on the Chief Duty Officer watchbill instead of going back to being an Emergency Vehicle Operator, or EVO. I had my reasons. For starters, my EVO license will have expired by the time I come back. Second, I've been at the command for four years now and lastly, there is precedent of me gaining this qualification in Iwakuni.

More good news, I built my ribbon rack with the projected ribbons and medals I earned while here. Holy cow! I'm onto my sixth row of ribbons. That of course made me feel even more accomplished.

Then to put the icing on the cake, I had a very good conversation with HM2 Yani Lopez, my work wife. My birthday was five days ago, but it seems like forever. Our replacements were supposed to arrive last night, but it seems like that has been pushed to tomorrow now.

I just shared what I had of the screenplay with HM3 Wes Alden, and he was mildly upset that there wasn't more to read. Again, felt good.

Postscript: This was the fruits of my labor beginning to ripen around the same time. All of those investments were beginning to pay off, and that was a good feeling at the time. When I left America for the first time in 2009 to go to Japan, I had exactly two ribbons. Like any clueless Sailor, I flew an international flight while in uniform. My poor mother, on the morning I left the house, she looked at my chest candy and sayid, "You only have two ribbons?" Unintentionally, it scared me into a ribbon chasing hound. I was proud to earn what I have because chest candy can tell a very good story.

30 Aug 20
Day 195

It was a lazy day, albeit it came with news worth writing about. My morning started like any other post-duty day except that I showered in the morning instead of late last night. The workload is well-paired like the weather these days in that there has been a noticeable drop. This entire week, the temperature has not been projected to get to 100 degrees. The evenings are actually very enjoyable. Tonight, I sat outside for two hours just talking. Then again, the company you keep is a huge difference maker.

So, the big news of the day was my roommate told me his Red Cross Message came through and he's leaving tomorrow to begin his journey back home. The intent is to make sure he is home in time to be with his wife for the birth of his first child, a boy they have agreed to name Henry. I'm very happy for Drumheller and his wife Ashley. I consider myself fortunate to live with him and he definitely made the deployment much more bearable than it could have been. I am indebted to knowing him, and dare I say, I will actually miss him and will depart calling him my friend.

Also watched *Now You See Me 2* (2016) and thought it was okay. I did see *Mission Impossible: Fallout* (2018) too last night. That was a movie that should have been seen in theaters.

Postscript: The fellowship was breaking. Of the new fathers on the deployment, everyone was able to be present for the birth except for HM2 Slagel and me. They were either able to leave early like my roommate or get home just in time after this was all over. Drumheller was an interesting guy who I will look back on with fond memories. He was a great sounding board for my problems, and there were always plenty of them to share, but he was just an agreeable guy. I'll never forget writing a letter to his mother explaining how good of a man she raised, and if there was one thing I was thankful for, it was to be living with him.

31 Aug 2020
Day 196

Well, it was time to say goodbye. Justin Drumheller, my roommate since May 12, has departed. He left the barracks for the last time in a van about 10 minutes ago. I wish him the best.

I wish my day would have been a better one, but I clearly woke up on the wrong side of the bed. Man! I was such a grouch when I came into work. Even though HM1 LaPenna was throwing some shade and stoking the fire, poking the bear or whatever else will have you, I know I didn't exactly need to be such the grump I was.

Anyway, I came in to brush up on the Transfer of Authority speech that PS2 Robert Krombach asked me to be the Master of Ceremonies for. We have our first rehearsal tomorrow. Our relieving unit came in today.

With the turnover official on September 6. I have two more days of duty remaining for the Pharmacy.

I switched my hospital duty day for the third of September. I'll be spending a lot of time at the hospital this next week, but that's okay with me because one day this war is going to end.

Had weigh-ins for the Biggest Loser competition. I gained two pounds, but I supposedly also gained muscle mass and I lost body fat percentage. Although not enough to matter.

Heard back from HM1 Whicker. Maybe I'll take more leave initially than I previously thought.

Postscript: HM1 LaPenna was generally not the confrontational type of guy. His "throwing shade" was more me not being in a mood to take jokes. PS2 Krombach, an entire chapter could be saved for this guy! He was about my age but had a full life when it came to time in the military. He started out working as an aviation guy on the USS Kitty Hawk when it was still commissioned. There is a good reason why its nickname at the end was the "Shitty Kitty." He then separated from active duty to join the National Guard, but came back in as a Personnelman, or PS. He was our enlisted administration officer, and if he were reading this, he'd be letting me know everything he did. Truth be told, it was a lot; unlike me he reported to work every single day. As of this publication, he is now a Master-at-Arms, or MA, keeping the Navy safe and secure. He was tasked with making the Change of Authority ceremony happen, and you could hear the stress coming from him. I'm glad he stepped up because it was a burden I'm sure no one wanted. HM1 Whicker retorted with a bit of reality, and it simply rubbed me the wrong way. Like most conflicts, allowing your ego to run wild is generally the first place to look for resolution.

1 Sept 2020
Day 197

So it begins. Today marked the first day of the MAP, or Meritorious Advancement Program, cycle. Some commands did not waste any time. A good example was Naval Hospital 29 in Palms, CA, where they called

HM3 [Redacted] up to the first paygrade that matters, HM2. Very proud of him. It was fun seeing his journey while we were together. His uncertainties and doubts. Not that I took pleasure in his pain; he showed his humanity.

It was a busy day. Three officers were promoted, and one of them was the pharmacist, now CDR Vince Deguzman. I let myself down by forgetting all about it! I tried to make up for it by writing a congratulatory note. He asked me if I wrote him a love letter and I replied with, one that went as far as the fraternization policy would permit.

It was stupid busy today. I could only call home for like two minutes before it was back on the grind. Pharmacy's replacement, SGT Bryan Sanchez is back and works full-time in the pharmacy. Until our Transfer of Authority ceremony on September 6, the Whiskey Pharmacy is doing all it can to make Sanchez's life easy after we leave.

Today was a big concentration on the Controlled Substance Inventory Board. Of course, there were discrepancies, and of course I had a hand in that, but I had a bigger hand in figuring out the solutions too, and that felt good. Earned my paycheck.

Postscript: Sergeant Sanchez was synonymous with making anyone's lives better. Never had a bad conversation with him, always performed, and when needed most, he appears like a guardian angel. It was because of his attitude and our familiarization with him that we wanted to make as good of a transition as possible. That included a lot of paperwork, which we were happy to do because it was for the type of guy who was following us.

2 Sept 2020
Day 198

It is becoming more like we are getting closer to the top of the roller coaster. This is exciting because today was much less stressful than yesterday. There seems to be a feeling of freedom in the air or something.

Woke up a little earlier than normal so we, the enlisted, could hold a working party. We emptied out a bunch of medications in the pharmacy that we are giving to a local Afghan hospital. Made us feel good, I'm sure.

The arrival of SGT Sanchez, I think, is coming at a critical time because it is my feeling that we are beginning to wear on one another. That's rich because we are so close to leaving, but when you're with a small enough group of folks in a small enough space for a long enough time, you begin to take note of behavior patterns.

Anyway, I cleaned my pistol today. It was dirty when I started, and I guess still dirty enough to fail by the standard set by HM1 Wilson. Luckily, it's going to the Air Force.

Then I went home and something that was never done, I turned the temperature up on the air-conditioning. I was able to call home and talk to Saori for an hour, but the best part was seeing Ollie wake up. First time for that!

Postscript: When the coronavirus came onto the scene, the pharmacy wasted no time or expense preparing for the worst. We had an enormous surplus of medications, which ended up never being used. To be fair, no one knew how bad it was going to be, and luckily it never came close to what we prepared for. There were many World War Z jokes going around at this time. Still, we had to get rid of all these medications, and we found an acceptor. Moving everything was another story, we had a caravan of pickup trucks to assist. Even the Romanian Army stopped by to help out. As a pharmacy tech, it was nice to see such a large, collective movement of help because this was a job that would have otherwise taken me a month to accomplish.

4 Sept 2020
Day 199 & 200

What a crummy past couple of days. The highlight was easily HM3 Wes Alden being meritoriously promoted to the next higher paygrade. So we had a cigar to celebrate.

Before that, straight personal hell. It was my hospital duty day, last one of mine for the deployment, and there was not one redeeming part of duty. Well, I did get to work with LT Simon Prado, and I have always gotten along with him rather well.

The night prior I watched the Sam Mendes movie *1917* (2019) and enjoyed it. The more I thought about it though the more unrealistic it was. I went to sleep around 0130, but instead of waking up at 0800 like a normal workday, it was 0600. Needless to say, I was tired for most of the day. Biking into work that early though, I noticed how cool it was, and it felt awesome.

When I was at work, because I was simply there, I was tasked with some pharmacy things. This of course aggravated me, so I hid most of the day in the supply warehouse. The problem with duty is it spans the entire workday, and the breaks between chores aren't really long enough to do anything else. After the last job I went home and quickly fell asleep. Woke up to both get dinner and smoke that cigar with Alden and went back to bed.

I looked at my journal, but my head hurt too much. YouTubed for half an hour and went to sleep. Despite sleeping over 8 hours, and rather deeply, I woke up with my headache. Got to work, showered, and began my day. I was in a solemn mood for a lot of the day. I just wanted to work and not be very social.

Of course, I was thinking about what would fix the itch I was having, and I think it was figured out. I'm now in the depression phase of not being selected for MAP from my own command. Even though I know my chances were slim, I know this was my best chance yet. Luckily, I tried telling Saori about it and she was very loving and supportive. I told her that if I was given the option to look for another job, I would.

These are the days I'm filled with so much doubt, and it hurts. Speaking of pain, a flight itinerary came in to get back to Japan, and it's not good. They have me flying out of Seattle, WA, all the way to Iwakuni. This is problematic on a couple of levels because I'm supposed to be flying from

Qatar to Japan and ROM (Restriction of Movement aka 14-day quarantine) in Atsugi. I forwarded what I knew to Master Chief Branch. Maybe and hopefully it will change, but at least I now have a flight home and unless they say, "This is the way" or "I have spoken," then I will live with that.

By the end of the workday, I was feeling better. HM1 LaPenna offered to take my pharmacy duty tonight if I honestly felt like I was going to get a promotable evaluation so I could go home and cry. I did not take him up on his generous offer.

Postscript: Surprisingly this is an entry that I feel needs little explanation. In looking at a map, the flight itinerary had me flying around the world in the "opposite" direction. This would only make my travel even longer to get home. This was because of COVID. Qatar International Airport was essentially shut down and so were most other international flights. Unless you flew into Japan on a military flight, you weren't coming in at all. That was what happened. I'll never forget what HM1 LaPenna did for me, and he probably would have taken my duty too had I been weak and cowardly enough to think so. This is a good demonstration of a burden of leadership because he knew how I ranked at the evaluation board but could not say anything until it was official. Hospital duty was different from pharmacy duty. We had to refill the water depots, go get the food, drop off the laundry, and then do all of that in reverse. It was easy work, but just made for a long day.

6 Sept 2020
Day 202

Odd timing to write this, but I swear I have my reasons. Technically it's 0100 on September 7, but I was busy.

There have been too many big dates I have missed on the day it actually happened in this journal, and for a variety of reasons too. Today was the Transfer of Authority ceremony to the Army. This marks the first "deployment is over" false-finishers for the time back to Sasebo. You know, that place all my babies are at.

As the Master of Ceremonies, I was met with praise afterward, but I always think the job could have been done better. There were a good number of Army awards given, none of them which were for me, but I am actually surprisingly okay with that. Maybe because I work with CDR Deguzman, who after earning his equivalent to the Navy Commendation Medal, went back to work immediately following the ceremony. To say that he was a hard worker is a gross understatement and borderline insulting to his effort, character, and poise. There is a lot to aspire to in terms of adopting his humility and grit.

The typhoon is now in Sasebo. I'd be lying if I said I wasn't nervous. Saori will report at daylight. Started watching a documentary on a guy who was eaten by a grizzly bear. Mail Call tomorrow.

Postscript: The Transfer of Authority ceremony was a shell of what it could have been, and that was because of COVID mitigations. All the distinguished guests were sat in chairs, spaced out, and the enlisted were way in the back and in close formation. As the master of ceremonies, I had to quickly adapt to a squeaky microphone that sat right behind the keynote speaker, the Brigadier General of the entire area of operations. I was hot, but so was everyone else. There were, I believe, 13 bronze star recipients from Victor Rotation. Whiskey had one, the Commanding Officer. Make of that what you will; some decisions I'll never be able to understand or, more importantly, accept.

8 Sept 2020
Day 203 & 204

It was nothing short of a wild and crazy two days, and my day is about to get much longer.

We began this tale in a sprint of action yesterday afternoon when the message came out that Whiskey staff with a last name beginning A through P would be leaving the next day. I don't think the halls were as abuzz when a mass casualty came in and we darted to the hospital.

Later in the night we had a final bonfire. For me, it was filled with delightful talk, again, with HM3 James Writer and HM2 [Redacted]. I always enjoyed talking to those two cats. The party was cut short when word started to spread around that there was an explosion at the burn pit. Luckily, it was just one patient, and he was ambulatory, but of course we feared and prepared for the worst.

When I got back to the barracks, I smoked another cigar and talked until 2230 outside. When I came in, I was too tired for anything besides YouTube, but was asleep before midnight.

The next day got wild from the beginning. At 0800 we had our End of Tour award ceremony. I had earned a NAM, or Navy Achievement Medal. It was short of my goal of a Navy Commendation Medal, but at this point I'm more focused on getting home. Is it bad to have such lofty goals? Probably not, provided the disappointment can be properly managed.

HM1 Wilson made a bad joke that maybe my command is waiting to MAP me when I get back. I don't want to even think about such pie in the sky ideas. That said, maybe that is still an option.

Afterwards, I putted around the pharmacy and learned in an email that I am in fact flying to Iwakuni where I will be bused and ROM in Sasebo after all. This is great news, but sad at the same time, especially if I won't be able to ROM at home but the barracks instead.

When I did get home, I took a nap and woke up to call home. I'm trying to apply the lessons read in the *Seven Principles for Making Marriage Work*. I think some strategies are helping, especially when Saori wants to talk about things I really don't care to.

Then during dinner, the bomb was dropped. Not only are we leaving tomorrow, but our showtime at the airport is 0330. Our working party begins at 0200.

I'm writing this entry at the laundromat, where so many postings here have been made in the past, and when I finish, I will start the final push to pack my last bags. Honestly, there really isn't a lot of time to reflect on my time here, especially within these pages. All I know is that I'm happy to leave and I won't even wish to come back.

As my final moment at the Role III hospital, I wrote a parting letter for my appreciation of getting to know Freddie from supply. I never got to learn his last name, but I will miss him the most.

Postscript: This was a wild time. Information was coming out at an alarming pace, and you had to be certain that what you were hearing was accurate. Our primary tool for mass communication was WhatsApp, and it was hopping at this time. Because Drumheller had left by this point, I had the room to myself; meaning that it fell on me to get a good checkout done. This was fine until they said they wanted the room to look a very specific way, and that took some maneuvering to do. Lots of laundry, and not a lot of sleep was the prescribed order of business. I remember leaving my bike on the bike rack for the next person to come along needing a ride.

FREDDIE

There exists a shortlist of people who have affected my life more than others while on this deployment, and Freddie is among them. I am not sure what made me gravitate to him, but for every question I had, he had a moment to explain an answer. Not all pearls of wisdom were applicable, but he taught me more about how to just chip away at a problem than anyone else I've ever met.

One of my first memories was trying to use the Swole 3 gym in the back of the hospital. He'd walk by chanting some encouraging words. In the supply warehouse there was a pushup box where you could rearrange your arm position to attack different parts of the chest, arms, and back. He pledged that he'd match whatever I did. When I was down and feeling sorry for myself, he'd give me space. I'd try to apologize, but he'd quickly dismiss my polite excuses and tell me that when I'm ready to work he'd be there. This went on for weeks, and he never lost faith in me.

The deployment was around the same time as the George Floyd debacle in Minnesota, and we'd have very good, objective discussions about race and inequality. He helped open up my world view with the insight of a black man. He was from Georgia, and I was from Wisconsin. Somehow, we met in the middle and I had a better understanding of his position and what Black Lives Matter meant because I had believed up until then that All Lives Mattered.

Freddie came to work every day, something I didn't do. It was something I was a bit ashamed about because there were some people who grinded each and every day on that deployment. Sure, I wasn't a contractor like him, and I wasn't getting paid like he was, but a deployment to Afghanistan was such an honor, and I feel like I failed at some point. Freddie only had an encouraging word and little story to help put things into perspective. I would find out why he was so damn big, he was a practice squad cornerback with the Dallas Cowboys, having played with the likes of Deion Sanders. To be at that level you have to have some intrinsic motivation. He went on to retire as a Captain in the Army and took a job as a contractor afterward.

Some people walk in and out of your life and that is what they are supposed to do. Freddie walked into my life and made a home within my heart, which will be with me forever. Thank you, Freddie, wherever you are, and I hope one day we meet again.

Part III:
Coming Home

9 Sept 2020
Day 205

I was three days shy of being in Afghanistan for four total months. In some way I feel cheated by the coronavirus and everything that it changed. On the other hand, I'm glad I'm not there anymore. I don't feel like Frodo did when his journey was complete. I feel like this is the end of a lifelong series of hills for me to climb.

Because I was the "weapons watch," I got to see how a military airport operates as they stacked luggage. My job was to make sure no one stole a gun, and its selling perk was I'd be the first Whiskey Sailor to board the plane. I was already asleep when everyone else came onboard.

A three-and-a-half-hour flight later we were in Kuwait. We were riding in a C-17, and the plane had multiple stops and cargo let alone its passengers. We were just along for the ride. Kuwait placed what I thought hot was on another level. It looked like some bombed bunkers from Desert Storm remained untouched, like a memorial, but they looked operational. Afterward, same plane, different cargo, and a one-hour flight to Qatar.

They had much needed Pizza Hut waiting for us. There were a lot of seabag drags today. We finally got through the airport whose security was charitable to put nicely and into "T Town" we went. These are open bay barracks that are designed to hold us for three days as we process out of this deployment and rotate back to home.

At the most we'll be here for 10 days. My pen is beginning to die. How poetic. I logged into the free Wi-Fi, told my family I was safe, and went to sleep from 1700-0220. Will talk about Qatar tomorrow, but it's humid.

Postscript: It was a mad dash to get the hell out of Kandahar. Not that the base was under attack and there was an evacuation, but everything up to this point was on such a short timeline. It felt really good to finally leave the country of Afghanistan. With that said, moving a unit as efficiently as possible is not an easy process. There is a bunch of hurrying up to wait, and you really do need patience to let the process happen.

I'll never forget how hot it was in Kuwait. As they were reloading the cargo, we stepped off the airplane to stretch our legs in a hangar and the breath was just taken from me. Qatar was just as hot as Kuwait, or so it seemed, but at this point we didn't even care. The caring about being stuck here would come later.

10 Sept 2020
Day 206

First day with a new pen. Let's see how it fairs, but, for a brief history lesson, it was this style of pen I originally wanted to use years ago when I bought this actual journal. There's a little cubby pocket in the back where I housed a few of these Pilot Precise V5 rolling pens with the extra fine tip. It now gets its debut.

Night two of Qatar is just as hot and humid as last night, but less of a surprise. Where I thought I would sleep deep into the night, it was about 2030, or 3.5 hours after going to bed. It would be safe to fear that my sleep schedule will become a beast of its own.

I don't do anything to exert myself. I lay in bed and get up only when I have to use the restroom, or if my back and hips demand it. On the Kindle I'm currently tearing up Mike Rowe's *That's the Way I Heard It*, a line which *The Thirsty Camel* ripped from. It's good, and in a world where I'm trying to limit phone use, especially YouTube, I'm finding a huge uptick in my reading, and that is good.

Today we signed our evaluations. As I expected, I earned an EP, or early promote, rating, the highest tier possible. Because it did not explicitly say I was the #1, my guess is someone else's did, but I'd rather not know who that could be. I need to convince myself that I can be satisfied with what I earned. That is one thing I can say; I do feel that score was earned. There were 20 Second Class Petty Officers who were ranked. Four had EP, 8 with MP (must-promote), and 8 were promotable.

We all got the same End of Tour Award, except one, who was the first ranked MP. I'm okay with that because it's time to go home.

Postscript: It's funny rereading what I write sometimes. Saying that "I'm okay with it," as if I am the final judge of another Sailor's performance. Like I had an all-seeing globe to tell me who was worthy and who wasn't. I knew I was in the running, but I did not think it was expected. It was a goal to have earned the EP, but something like that just isn't expected. What I believe I was trying to tell myself was I simply was over the deployment and ready to come home and get back to my life. The goals were either accomplished or not. It was merely the waiting game from here, and it was as difficult as it could have been.

EVALUATION REPORT & COUNSELING RECORD (E1-E6)

RCS BUPERS 1610-1

1. Name (Last, First MI Suffix)	2. Rate	3. Desig	4. SSN
RASTALL, CALVIN W	HM2	SW/AW	

5. ACT	FTS	INACT	AT/ADSW/265	6. UIC	7. Ship/Station	8. Promotion Status	9. Date Reported
X				3952A	NATO ROLE 3 MMU	REGULAR	20FEB18

Occasion for Report: 10. Periodic [ ] 11. Detachment of Individual [X] 12. Promotion/Frocking [ ] 13. Special [ ]

Period of Report: 14. From: 20FEB18 15. To: 20SEP10

16. Not Observed Report [ ] Type of Report: 17. Regular [ ] 18. Concurrent [X]

20. Physical Readiness

21. Billet Subcategory (if any): INDIV AUG

22. Reporting Senior (Last, FI MI)	23. Grade	24. Desig	25. Title	26. UIC	27. SSN
	CAPT	2100	CO	3952A	

28. Command employment and command achievements.

Forward deployed to NATO Role 3 Multinational Medical Unit, Kandahar, Afghanistan, providing world class combat trauma care in support of RESOLUTE SUPPORT MISSION and OPERATION FREEDOM'S SENTINEL.

29. Primary/Collateral/Watchstanding duties. (Enter primary duty abbreviation in box.)

PHARMACY TECH PRI: Pharmacy Technician, Pharmacy Department-4. COLL: Command PAO Member-4; Command Diversity Committee-4; Command Training Team-6; Department Mail Orderly-4. WATCH: Command Duty-4; Pharmacy-4. TEMADD: ECRC/NEMTI/NIACT 20FEB18-20APR26.

For Mid-term Counseling Use. (When completing EVAL, enter 30 and 31 from counseling worksheet and sign 32.)	30. Date Counseled	31. Counselor	32. Signature of Individual Counseled
	NOT REQ		

PERFORMANCE TRAITS: 1.0 - Below standards/not progressing or UNSAT in any one standard; 2.0 - Does not yet meet all 3.0 standards; 3.0 - Meets all 3.0 standards; 4.0 - Exceeds most 3.0 standards; 5.0 - Meets overall criteria and most of the specific standards for 5.0. Standards are not all inclusive.

PERFORMANCE TRAITS	1.0* Below Standards	2.0 Progressing	3.0 Meets Standards	4.0 Above Standards	5.0 Greatly Exceeds Standards
33. PROFESSIONAL KNOWLEDGE: Technical knowledge and practical application. NOB [ ]	-Marginal knowledge of rating, specialty or job. -Unable to apply knowledge to solve routine problems. -Fails to meet advancement/PQS requirements. [ ]	[ ]	-Strong working knowledge of rating, specialty and job. -Reliably applies knowledge to accomplish tasks. -Meets advancement/PQS requirements on time. [ ]	[X]	- Recognized expert, sought out by all for technical knowledge. - Uses knowledge to solve complex technical problems. - Meets advancement/PQS requirements early/with distinction. [ ]
34. QUALITY OF WORK: Standard of work; value of end product. NOB [ ]	-Needs excessive supervision. -Product frequently needs rework. -Wasteful of resources. [ ]	[ ]	-Needs little supervision. -Produces quality work. Few errors and resulting rework. -Uses resources efficiently. [ ]	[ ]	- Needs no supervision. - Always produces exceptional work. No rework required. - Maximizes resources. [X]
35. COMMAND OR ORGANIZATIONAL CLIMATE/EQUAL OPPORTUNITY: Contributing to growth and development, human worth, community. NOB [ ]	-Actions counter to Navy's retention/reenlistment goals. -Uninvolved with mentoring or professional development of subordinates. -Actions counter to good order and discipline and negatively affect Command/Organizational climate. -Demonstrates exclusionary behavior. Fails to value differences from cultural diversity. [ ]	[ ]	-Positive leadership supports Navy's increased retention goals. Active in decreasing attrition. -Actions adequately encourage/support subordinates' personal/professional growth. -Demonstrates appreciation for contributions of Navy personnel. Positive influence on Command climate. -Values differences as strengths. Fosters atmosphere of acceptance/inclusion per EO/EEO policy. [ ]	[X]	- Measurably contributes to Navy's increased retention and reduced attrition objectives. - Proactive leader/exemplary mentor. Involved in subordinates' personal development leading to professional growth/sustained commitment. - Initiates support programs for military, civilian, and families to achieve exceptional Command and Organizational climate. - The model of achievement. Develops unit cohesion by valuing differences as strengths. [ ]
36. MILITARY BEARING/CHARACTER: Appearance, conduct physical fitness, adherence to Navy Core Values. NOB [ ]	-Consistently unsatisfactory appearance. -Poor self-control, conduct resulting in disciplinary action. -Unable to meet one or more physical readiness standards. -Fails to live up to one or more Navy Core Values: HONOR, COURAGE, COMMITMENT. [ ]	[ ]	-Excellent personal appearance. -Excellent conduct conscientiously complies with regulations. -Complies with physical readiness program. -Always lives up to Navy Core Values: HONOR, COURAGE, COMMITMENT. [ ]	[X]	- Exemplary personal appearance. - Model of conduct, on and off duty. - A leader in physical readiness. - Exemplifies Navy Core Values: HONOR, COURAGE, COMMITMENT. [ ]
37. PERSONAL JOB ACCOMPLISHMENT/INITIATIVE: Responsibility, quantity of work. NOB [ ]	-Needs prodding to attain qualification or finish job. -Prioritizes poorly. -Avoids responsibility. [ ]	[ ]	-Productive and motivated. Completes tasks and qualifications fully and on time. -Plans/prioritizes effectively. -Reliable, dependable, willingly accepts responsibility. [ ]	[ ]	- Energetic self-starter. Completes tasks or qualifications early, far better than expected. - Plans/prioritizes wisely and with exceptional foresight. - Seeks extra responsibility and takes on the hardest jobs. [X]

1. Name (Last, First MI Suffix)	2. Rate	3. Desig	4. SSN
RASTALL, CALVIN W	HM2	SW/AW	[redacted]

PERFORMANCE TRAITS	1.0* Below Standards	2.0 Progressing	3.0 Meets Standards	4.0 Above Standards	5.0 Greatly Exceeds Standards
38. TEAMWORK: Contributions to team building and team results. NOB [ ]	-Creates conflict, unwilling to work with others, puts self above team. -Fails to understand team goals or teamwork techniques. -Does not take direction well. [ ]	- [ ]	-Reinforces others' efforts, meets commitments to team. -Understands goals, employs good teamwork techniques. -Accepts and offers team direction. [ ]	[ ]	-Team builder, inspires cooperation and progress. -Focuses goals and techniques for teams. -The best at accepting and offering team direction. [X]
39. LEADERSHIP: Organizing, motivating and developing others to accomplish goals. NOB [ ]	-Neglects growth/development or welfare of subordinates. -Fails to organize, creates problems for subordinates. -Does not set or achieve goals relevant to command mission and vision. -Lacks ability to cope with or tolerate stress. -Inadequate communicator. -Tolerates hazards or unsafe practices. [ ]	- [ ]	-Effectively stimulates growth/development in subordinates. -Organizes successfully, implementing process improvements and efficiencies. -Sets/achieves useful, realistic goals that support command mission. -Performs well in stressful situations. -Clear, timely communicator. -Ensures safety of personnel and equipment. [ ]	[X]	-Inspiring motivator and trainer, subordinates reach highest level of growth and development. -Superb organizer, great foresight, develops process improvements and efficiencies. -Leadership achievements dramatically further command mission and vision. -Perseveres through the toughest challenges and inspires others. -Exceptional communicator. -Makes subordinates safety-conscious, maintains top safety record. -Constantly improves the personal and professional lives of others. [ ]

40. Individual Trait Avg. total of trait scores divided by number of graded traits.	41. I recommend this individual for (maximum of two): Assignment in Rating, Sea Special Programs, Shore Special Programs, Commissioning Programs, Special Warfare Programs, Rating Instructor Duty, Other. (Be specific)	42. Signature of Rater (Typed Name & Rate): I have evaluated this member against the above performance standards and have forwarded written explanation of marks 1.0 and 5.0.
4.43	LPO AT SEA / OCS	[signature] WINK, C J, HMCS Date: 10Sep 20

43. COMMENTS ON PERFORMANCE: * All 1.0 marks, three 2.0 marks, and 2.0 marks in Block 35 must be specifically substantiated in comments. Comments must be verifiable. Font must be 10 or 12 Pitch (10 or 12 point) only. Use upper and lower case.

*** HIGH CALIBER SAILOR WHO PUTS THE MISSION FIRST. MORE THAN READY FOR PO1! ***

- MISSION ORIENTED. Filled, reviewed, & dispensed 3.5K prescriptions and sterile products for 13 providers who provided trauma care & force health protection for 8,500 NATO warfighters; contributed to the successful execution of 2 MASCALs, 43 trauma cases, 111 surgical procedures, & the management of 3K line-items worth $3M with no discrepancies.
- ASTUTE MANAGER. Supply PO, maintained 550 line-items including 60 controlled substances worth $855K. Managed Reverse Distribution Program, returned credit of $55K. Developed & sustained COVID-19 pharmaceutical supply chain, resulted in zero shortages and sustained optimal operational readiness. Implemented FDA extension of 51 line-items, saving $7K.
- CMD INVOLVED. PAO editor, led 4 enlisted & advised 2 officers; produced 8 articles for friends/families. Diversity Committee, assisted in 3 focus groups & supported the Navy's "Diversity & Inclusion" initiative; fostered Navy EO policy objectives. Master of Ceremony for the 122nd HM Birthday celebration & Transfer of Authority ceremony; displayed sense of heritage. Sailor of the Month board member & validated 2 Lean Six Sigma projects; streamlined supply chain processes & access to care. PSG RSCA: 3.96.

*** HAS EARNED MY HIGHEST RECOMMENDATION FOR PROMOTION! ***

44. QUALIFICATIONS/ACHIEVEMENTS - Education, awards, community involvement, etc., during this period.

QUAL: NEC (3). AWD: NA; ACM; AFSM; NATO; SSDR; Sailor of the Month; Motivator of the Month; LOA (2). EDU: Bachelor's Degree; NRTC (3); EPME (8); Non-GMT (8).

Promotion Recommendation	NOB	Significant Problems	Progressing	Promotable	Must Promote	Early Promote	47. Retention: Not Recommended [ ] Recommended [X]
45. INDIVIDUAL						X	48. Reporting Senior Address
46. SUMMARY	X	0	0	8	8	4	BUMED 7700 ARLINGTON BLVD STE 5113 FALLS CHURCH, VA 22042

49. Signature of Senior Rater (Typed Name & Grade/Rate): I have reviewed the evaluation of this member against these performance standards and have provided written explanation to support the marks of 1.0 and 5.0.	50. Signature of Reporting Senior
[signature] DEGUZMAN, V E, CDR Date: 7 SEP 20	[signature] Date: 6 SEP 2020 Summary Group Average: 3.97

51. Signature of Individual Evaluated. "I have seen this report, been apprised of my performance, and understand my right to submit a statement."	52. Typed name, grade, command, UIC, and signature of Regular Reporting Senior on Concurrent Report
I intend to submit a statement [ ] I do not intend to submit a statement [X] Cal Rastall Date: 10SEP20	ALSINA, M F, CAPT NMRTU SASEBO, 35274 Date:

11 Sept 2020
Day 207

Never forget. It's been 19 years since the World Trade Center towers came down. Had they not, there is a very real chance I either never would have wanted to go to Afghanistan, or maybe know anything about it outside of *Rambo III* (1988). So yes, it's strongly linked between this date and where I am. Everyone in my era who joined any branch of the armed services wished they could have gotten the chance to come here. As the last rotation of Role III, I'm actually humbled by the chance I had to get into the fight and do my part. I didn't kick down doors, pop smoke, go high speed, or low drag, but I played a role in a much larger band. Maybe one day I will fully believe that.

As I write, it's 0400 on the 12th. I became too cold in the barracks and woke up to warm up, but the humidity is almost comedic. I really don't know how to describe it. For now, it's better than being in the frigid barracks, which have their place during the day, but worked a little too well tonight.

Called home to Saori, I had a mind lapse because at 1700 in Qatar for some reason I thought it would have been 2100 in Japan and I could catch the boys before bedtime. Well, it was actually 2300, and I was able to have a good conversation for about 40 minutes with Mrs. Rastall. Oliver continued a family tradition and was circumcised today.

Finished the *Seven Principles of Marriage* and the Mike Rowe book. Onto the devilish *48 Laws of Power.*

Postscript: To be honest, there are plenty of people who join the military across a wide spectrum of reasons. Kicking Osama's ass is not the end-all reason. Some people just wanted their tuition paid for. That is an important distinction from saying "free college" because nothing we do while serving is free. I'm a firm believer that the benefits veterans receive are earned with interest. Some people simply had no other option and needed a way to support their families. So no, my mother taught me better than to speak in absolutes, but in the context of the day it was written, after where I had just been, it seemed the most appropriate thing to say. Marriage is something that takes a lot of work, many books are written about that, and I see nothing shameful for talking about wanting to keep that axe sharp.

12 Sept 2020
Day 208

This was a rather forgettable day for me. Maybe the best part was calling home and getting to hear Saori vent about the boys. Atticus especially is being extra naughty and Josiah is being extra rough on his middle brother. Ollie is just hanging out, taking up an extra arm. In other words, the Rastall boys need their Papa home pronto, Tonto.

Alas, I am here, in "T Town," where the only good thing is all the time to read. That's the end of my list. I don't know when I'm flying out, I don't like lining up to be led outside the gate like cattle and load a couple packed buses to the galley, and I don't like the scarcity of chairs.

A huge majority of my day is spent on my back, literally. It's hotter here than Afghanistan, the capacity is filling up and the air-conditioning is set so low, I need to wake up at night and walk around outside to warm up. Anyway, I did a load of laundry and took a shower, but not in that order.

Maybe what I'm trying to say is I'm beginning to feel the first pangs of frustration. I know that "one day this war is going to end," but we are more than done; just let us go home! Food here is bland, nothing to write home about. Oh, I added a savings account to my USAA online banking, and I bought coffee that will be delivered straight to the clinic. Reorganized my Amazon account to align the 1-click purchase with my allowance fund. Only six more days of this. YouTube?

Postscript: Under "normal" circumstances, we would have only spent a couple of days in Qatar to be processed out of CENTCOM, or Central Command. We would then be flown to Germany to a retreat and take classes between beer binges to learn how to reintegrate with our families and society. Whiskey was not so fortunate. A lot of what we did was based on our own imagination.

13 Sept 2020
Day 209

Each day that passes here is more soul-sucking than the next, except for one thing here. The start of the NFL season kicked off, and the Packers have started off on the right foot. Although I left the game early to write this, it started at 2000, it was a lofty margin victory. Aaron Rodgers had over 300 yards in the air and passed four touchdowns. In any case it was an interesting setup because we were all pirating the streaming. None of us cared; we just wanted to watch football. More importantly, we just wanted something to take our minds off of this place.

I slept until 0930 or so, and went to go get lunch, but took another three-hour nap around noon. Woke up, kissed the boys goodnight, Japan is six hours ahead of us, and laid around in bed. As of this writing I have not read my book once today.

To that end, I did have a couple of meaningful conversations. The first one was with HM2 Jesse John. We were talking about our evaluations we signed a few days ago. Next was with the other two pharmacy techs, and it was more of the debrief after the debrief of evaluation signings. We jotted a lot of plotting for where it goes from here after we go home. I was appreciative they took the time to do that since it clearly wasn't required.

Saori sent a video of a clever Josiah sneaking into my office to watch Netflix and locking the door behind him.

Postscript: I will never forget Jake Wilson and Mike LaPenna. They would help me turn into what I would become. It has been written all over this book, and I'm proud that I was lucky enough to work so closely with them. Was every day a joyous affair? Absolutely not. With the best of times, come the worst of times? Hell yes. Were the lessons taught and heard? I want to think so.

16 Sept 2020
Day 210, 211 & 212

Finally a night where I can't sleep! It sounds weird to say that, but I'm "used" to not sleeping at night in Qatar. I fell asleep around 1730 today and woke up at 2030. Went outside and the usual suspects were sitting there. That is where our story begins.

For the past three or four nights a group of us has congregated around our little picnic table. We consist of LT Kevin Veatch, HM3 James Writer, HM2 Albert Terrell, and me. HM1 Michael LaPenna often joins up when he comes out to smoke (which is more often than anyone else by far on the deployment). What we choose to talk about is as endless as it is deep, and I love it.

HM3 Writer is, to me, the best storyteller of the whole lot. He's got either a very interesting life or a heck of a knack describing some boring stuff. Either way, I'm constantly left captivated with what he shares. Terrell and Veatch are excellent supporting characters and parry off one another. When I can, I try to jump in, but I'm just happy to listen to a voice that isn't my own from reading to myself. In no way could I compete with these juggernauts. If there was going to be one part of my time in Qatar 2.0 that I'll miss, it will be sharing that table with those guys.

That leads me to a hard truth, none of us seems to be preparing to say goodbye. Maybe it is because it seems like time is standing still here and we'll be together forever. Of course that is not true, but there is almost no posturing that once we hit Baltimore this will be all over.

I had a little taste of that in fact yesterday when I was in my rack minding my own business when all of a sudden HM2 Renardo Reid was like, "Pack your bags, all the overseas guys are leaving in an hour." I jumped from my bed, all excited saying delirious things like, "I am a respected member of a mid-western state!" Well, that kind of language went on for about 10 minutes as I was trying to figure out how to pack when the newly promoted Senior Chief Atangan came into our building and said that I wasn't going anywhere.

That's correct, everyone who was stationed overseas to include mainland Japan, Okinawa and Guam all left last night except me. In the midst of a lot of emotion was the discovery that I was the only person from overseas who had a full itinerary to go home. My journey will begin on the 19th like everyone else. With that said, I guess there was a scheduling problem for everyone who left, and they might actually get home after me. Classic tortoise and the hare situation. I haven't confirmed that rumor however, but it would certainly shore up the "everything happens for a reason" ideology.

My phone calls with Saori have been rather pleasant recently. There is a lot of me listening, mostly because I've had nothing newsworthy to share, and as long as I listen without interfering or "fixing" her problems, life is good. Today though she shared some bad news. Miyuki's doctors have reason to believe that her cancer has spread to her liver. More tests next week will confirm.

This is of course devastating to hear and I wish I could be there. Saori shared how surprised she was when she found out Miyuki is taking two doses of pain medication a day. Wondering what pain management is used for cancer patients in Japan, I asked what she was taking. "Aspirin" was what I was told, and I started laughing! Definitely a different care plan in the States.

CDR Vince Deguzman sent a picture of the Army Achievement Medal CENTCOM wrote for me. He asked for my command's address, and I went ahead and ordered my updated ribbon rack with that confirmation. One rack cost $36, and I bought two. Still happy I'm up to six rows now.

I decided when I get back to Sasebo that I will have two asks. First, I want to wear my service uniform everyday. After this deployment if I never have to wear cammies again I'll be happy. The second ask is to be put on the Chief Duty Officer watchbill. This'll be a much taller request. So much so that I dreamt I was arguing about it with my Leading Chief Petty Officer, or LCPO, as Master Chief Branch served as arbitrator. Either way, I've been spending a lot of time building my argument and envisioning counter-argument points.

Still reading *48 Laws of Power.* Some learning points and a lot of self-realization for finding how I behave with how I'm treated. I think it'll pair well with my book on stoicism I have lined up next.

Postscript: That was a wild day. Reid was stationed in Okinawa. I touched on our relationship previously, but at that moment he was my best friend. As it turned out, the "overseas group" did get home before us, but in the long run I'm happy I was left with the guys just a little bit longer. In the moment though, it was devastating, yet funny at the same time.

18 Sept 2020
Day 213 & 214

Greetings from the Fatherland. Correct, I am back out of the Middle East for the first time since April, and it feels good. It was also a beautiful 51 degrees outside. Couldn't be happier.

How did I get here? What was it like? We were going to have another absolutely boring day on the 17th. Nothing to say or write home about, except for one thing. The two Senior Chiefs, our original HMCS Cameron Wink and our newly selected HMCS Melvin Atanagan, bought pizza for the enlisted crew. This may not seem important, and the fact it was two hours late to arrive was all too familiar with the Navy. No, what I meant was there was a pang of the feeling amongst us as a group that this was it. The next day will begin our final descent to the breaking of our fellowship.

Of course I hold all the brotherly moments against the metric of *A River Runs Through It* (1992), especially the scene at the end where they caught their fish and were talking along the banks with their father. Some music in movies really do make or break a film, but I'm getting off track. The last time I felt that kinship was when we cut all those IV bags together. It's not a feeling which comes often.

So that night, we sat around our racks and told as many jokes and stories as we could. It was a delightful scene. I've decided to let everyone sign and inscribe my book from HM1 Wilson, *Stillness is the Key*. It filled up pretty good and I'm looking forward to reading it when we've separated.

Now, Sept 18 was a different story. Very jubilant, lots of excitement in the air. It could be felt, and everyone knew it. I didn't lay down at all after waking up, I was sick and tired of being on my back. Had a touching phone call from Japan. Josiah seemed engaged and even asked if one of my coworkers was "Uncle Max."

Then at 1800, the long march began. Packed our shit and made it to the airport. Lots of dragging seabags. Of course, as it's a very muggy 90 degrees at night in Qatar, it's an uncomfortable ordeal. Plus, we weren't alone; an Air Force unit was leaving with us, which made our lines longer and patience shorter.

For a flight that wasn't scheduled to depart until midnight, we waited until 0200. Some things just write themselves I swear. To that end, our flight was awesome, or as good as it could be. We flew in a 747 and the entire back of the plane had eight people. Needless to say, I had my own row to myself. That was convenient because I became extra sleepy after eating three hot meal courses. There were something like 150 souls on board and 400 meals.

Got a nice cramp in every joint I have from laying in an airplane row, but it was worth it. We have flown into Rammstein, Germany, and for an Air Force facility it's huge, and nice is an understatement. No alcohol here though, so it could be better. I mean, it is Germany after all.

Postscript: The seabag drags are the dumbest, yet most necessary part of traveling with a military unit. Generally an enlisted function, the officers who help the most get the most brownie points from "the boys." There were certainly some who helped more than others, and it showed in how they were treated. One of the biggest lessons learned was how much I overpacked, and how I won't be guilty of that next time. Other people, mostly officers, had close to 200 lb of luggage. I know this because we had a competition at the terminal when checking bags. And it said on our ticket. This does not include our issued gear either, the protective equipment like bulletproof vests and kevlar helmets.

19 Sept 2020
Day 215

This is a very important date to many of the Whiskey Rotation because their journey ended. They went home to their families, el fin, so to speak. The reservists and me, not so much. The rest of the overseas crew is now home.

To be fair and honest, this trip to Seattle so far was as nice as it could have been. It was eight hours at the airport before we flew to Germany from Qatar. It was a six-hour flight on a seemingly empty 747. We had a three-hour layover at Rammstein where I mostly slept through it, and then it was another eight-hour flight to Baltimore on the, again, mostly empty 747. My bags were seemingly one of the first off the baggage claim and the most unceremonious goodbye ever took place.

It was flying into BWI that I had my last hit of nicotine gum. It might hurt, but I've been here before and was expecting it. From BWI, it was a three-hour layover to get on the plane to Denver which was 3.5 hours. Denver Airport was a flash, I was there for less than an hour, but I was upgraded to business class for the first time in my life. It was 2.5 hours to Seattle, and I guess I was sitting next to my pilot for the Patriot Express flight on Monday. Didn't talk, slept the entire flight. Bags one of the first off the belt again, and took a shuttle to the hotel where that was a wrap for the day. It felt so nice to get my uniform off. I'm staying at the Holiday Inn Express and I am a big fan.

I mean, we didn't allow ourselves a proper goodbye. The fellowship is broken. It's a weird feeling, but I still don't consider myself home yet. Even when I get to Commander Fleet Activities Sasebo, I won't be home.

Hey, watching the Packers at 1000 is a cool feeling. #westcoast

Postscript: The last person I spoke to was Captain Daniel Kahler. We were just waiting for our bags. Other people were helping separate the luggage as it was coming off the belt, but I was too cool to help. When my bags came, I picked them up and left.

Senior Chief Cameron Wink said something to voice his approval for my help, but the deployment was over. I was too wrapped up in myself to care. I walked my issued gear to a designated rally point, dropped it off, and then walked around the airport to find my gate. Only there did an odd sense fall upon me, and I couldn't figure it out. It wasn't joy, shame, or an inward feeling. I was observing something but didn't know what I was seeing. Then it hit me, Baltimore's airport was damn near empty of travelers. It felt like walking into 28 Days Later *(2002). HM2 [Redacted] paid me back for the Denny's I bought him in California with my first* Big Mac *in months. There was one more observation. Wearing your uniform is a magnet for unwanted attention. Well, we had to travel in uniform, and if it had gotten me beer, I would have been happier, but it also gets us the fanfare of questions, "Where are you coming from?"* OR *hearing their stories of when they were in the service. Getting to Seattle was as easy as it could have been, albeit not in the most comfort. I knew there was a lot of road in front of me, but not sure how much it would turn out.*

20 Sept 2020
Day 216

It was actually a very nice farewell to America, and to all of this.

I woke up jet lagged and didn't actually sleep too much. Maybe it was because I was excited. There was one goal in mind, and that was to watch the Packer game. Because we were on the west coast, the game started at 1000. Perfect.

The front desk called me a taxi, and I assumed they told the dispatch where I wanted to go, a place called Twin Peaks. When the taxi arrived, there was an obvious disconnect. We settled on "any bar which plays football and is open." After a $31 cab fare, I arrived at a place nicely named The Spot.

It is your typical sports bar, and was a little out of place, but sat with some other Packer fans, Steve, and his son, Chase. The Packers won, and they won big. The conversation was good, and we decided to drive together to Twin Peaks after all. The second tab was $113. I pretty much had a beer in my hand from about 1030 until they dropped me off at my hotel at 1930. Very nice people and fortunate to have met them. They made my day and put Seattle in a good light.

Steve made me take his number. Although I don't know if I'll need it, I'm glad to have it. I went into one bar to watch the Packers and left with two friends. Not a bad return on investment.

After getting home, I went straight to bed. When I woke up at 0100 as planned, I wasn't feeling good, but I began laundry, which was way overpriced. Turns out the dryer sucked, and I didn't get fully dried clothes to pack. Left the hotel at 0330 and took the complimentary shuttle to the SEA-TAC airport. Boom!

Postscript: That was very nice of those two guys. I was absolutely intending to enjoy the game by myself, but it worked out. There was probably no way I looked like I was in the military, but the nice tan I had definitely implied that I had just been somewhere hot. Traveling by myself is a low-key thing I like to do. Not just because I get to meet people like the Steve & Chase, but because I like the planning and execution of getting from one place to the other with as little interference as possible except for my own complacency. I love my wife, she is the mother of my children and means a great deal to me, but there are times when throwing her off a bridge might be a better option. Traveling with her is usually one of those times.

23 Sept 2020
Day 217, 218 & 219

Sometimes I think God is a comedian even though I know he's everything at once. Just when I thought Qatar was the worst part of the deployment, and I hit my rock bottom, I'm thrown a shovel.

So here I am, thrown into the Sasebo barracks and this is my second night. I can't believe it's the 23rd of September. Clearly, I lost a day flying into Japan, but let's talk about the trip.

Realizing I'm on a government flight and many military families will be making the trip with me, I scrambled to find some ear plugs. Of course, they're not in my carry-on bag. Because it's a commercial flight and not a C-17 Air Force flight, complimentary ear plugs were not an option; I had to buy my own. To my chagrin, the only ones available were the $10.99 plastic kind. After being spoiled in Qatar with the foamies, even buying my own box from Amazon, these were the most ill-fitting for the most important flight! They hurt my ears and didn't do anything to keep the noise out.

Or did they? I saw one family with two sets of twins! No doubt they have an amazing story, but they were on my flight, so it evened out quickly.

To my surprise, the flight was only 10 hours and 45 minutes to Yokota, Japan. I slept a little, but mostly read. At the airport I overpaid for some random *Entertainment Weekly* special issue covering *The West Wing* (1999). Read it cover to cover. Then I tried to sink my teeth into the *What Women Want* book by Tucker Max I had started in Qatar, but I read 100 pages and felt like I hadn't gotten anywhere.

When we deplaned in Yokota, it was cute to see all the new Japan arrivals. Taking pictures of everything, trying to figure out conversion rates, etc. It reminded me of a young buck I once knew in 2009. I don't blame them. After a two-hour layover, we were back in the air.

It was only a 67-minute flight and I slept through most of it. Then Iwakuni and the start of my nightmare began. No lie, they were gowned up like we had Smallpox and Ebola combined. In my opinion we were treated almost like Lepers. It was a sight to behold, and we were off on the bus to Sasebo, another five-hour trip.

The only good thing Yani told me was her sponsoree was on the bus. I found her, HN Grace Gunning, and we talked for most of the trip. She's eager and left a good first impression. It was about 2200 when we rolled up to the barracks.

They told us our rooms were on the fifth floor. Because I only had one seabag and my carry-on with me, I was fine, but I saw the harrowing look in my cohort's eyes, they had EVERYTHING with them since most of them were transferring to Sasebo. They had to carry those bags up five flights of stairs. I guess the elevator wasn't suitable for Lepers like us. Of course I helped them. Sure got hot fast, though!

We were told the ridiculous rules too, which I found myself poking holes in the system even then. Eventually I went to bed, but not without counting my blessings that there was complimentary Wi-Fi and even chairs in our rooms! Never thought I'd be so happy.

The next day, today, there was a lot of lounging around. There were a couple of perks to the day though. My old friend HM1 (SW/AW) Brandon Schram called me from Atsugi. Very appreciative that he took the time to do that. Called Saori and took a nap. When I woke up, Zach Nebus called me to ask which room was mine. He sent a nice little care package, and I split half of it with Gunning.

Was more active on the SCPOA chat group since February. That felt good to be back there, chatting amongst peers I have known, but I could feel myself getting aggressive. Certainly a byproduct of my frustration. It was certainly mounting. Before I started this entry, I submitted the following Facebook status:

Yes, I'm back in Sasebo, but I can't accept I'm home until I can hold my babies again. To be honest, I'm mishandling the culture shock on a few different levels. Stick with me, I'll catch up to a COVID world soon enough. I've done more with less.

The amount of support was particularly endearing to read. It should be noted that a lion's share of that support came from the military friendships I have forged in Sasebo throughout the years. By now it's safe to say that most civilians I know are so in the dark on how to behave, act, or support the military, especially those deployed, that I can hardly get mad at them for their inability to relate or even empathize. I know they say "welcome home" or "stay safe" with a good heart, and I shouldn't expect more than that, but this experience has helped forge my outlook on how I will show my love and support to the troops in the future.

Postscript: This is a little hard to translate from my mind to paper. There was seemingly a larger sense amongst my extended family that I was gone than with my Japanese family. I think the primary reason why this happened was because I had already been "gone" from Wisconsin for so long already. I left for boot camp in 2008, and this was 2020. Of course, I'd pop in the motherland to visit from time to time, but especially with children, my returns home have become even more infrequent. To someone who never left, in a way it didn't matter where I was, I was not back in Wisconsin. It is hard to say "welcome back" when I was not in the same place. Japan has had to become my home away from home. Not that it is my first option, but it's certainly better than other places the Navy could send me.

24 Sept 2020
Day 220

Night three about to begin. Since I'm still jet lagged, I did a lion's share of the sleeping in the mid-afternoon before dinner and then some more after dinner. Woke up to the boys going to bed. Atticus was in pain it seemed, or he was faking something. Apparently, he told Saori his stomach hurt, and he did present signs of abdominal distress. Maybe he's just full of crap, literally.

Josiah is showing off his English comprehension more and more, and it's awesome. As far as days in quarantine, this might have been a better one. All the boxes from deployment, minus three which were at the house already, are now in my barracks room. I didn't know I had mailed so much stuff back, but it appears to all be intact.

The biggest gem is getting my computer back. I've almost immediately started transcribing my journal. Wow, I wrote a lot! Started doing some calisthenics in my room too. Didn't do too well, but it's a start.

There were a lot of care package deliveries too. Alesha Vine sent water and flavor packets, and so did Nichole Bonadie. Travon Martin threw in a pack of water too. Oh! Alesha also sent a 12-pack of Miller Light. I sent half of what I had to HN Gunning's room. One day she'll be networked, but for now, I feel that since I have the "high ground" then it's my responsibility to support how I can.

Called Iwakuni's air terminal and found out they have Gunning's luggage.

Postscript: I was never bored while in ROM. The idea itself was still so new to me. Restriction of Movement didn't exist when I left. Now I was stuck in a barracks room only 15 miles from my house where my family was. Because this could not be changed, I made up for lost time. Why was everything waiting for me at the post office? I am not sure because I spread it out across months. There it was, all together, and now it was in my room. The only thing I wasn't excited about was knowing I had to get it all downstairs and back home.

25 Sept 2020
Day 221

About to enter night four here. It's nice to have goals, and I consider myself lucky to have them.

Before that, I would like to mention here all the kind phone calls I've been getting. Brandon Schram and I have been talking more these past three days than the past five years combined, and I love it. Then yesterday I got a call from the former HM2, one Eric Allen. He's living a good life in Florida. Our call was something like a half hour long. He's always been a hoot to talk to and it was so nice to see him in a good place. I also got a nice message from Brandon Scott. We did a little catching up.

I've been at my computer trying to transcribe all these journal entries. It's a slow process. It gets even more daunting when I think how many times I'm going to be rereading my entries to revise and expand, and even longer when I index everything. Maybe it'll pay off, maybe for my own entertainment, but hopefully not.

Yani Lopez sent over a care package that was appreciated.

I wish I had more to share, but my day was really routine. I've been dreaming a lot. They aren't nightmares, but vivid enough to wake me up. Most times I can't fall back asleep. Not sure what that means. Another surprising habit or lack thereof is the amount of reading I've done. Perhaps transcribing is taking up my "awake" time.

Lots of YouTube though, but by now it's whatever.

Postscript: Eat, Sleep, Transcribe. That was my main job while I had the time to do it. Eric Allen was my sponsor to Sasebo back in 2017. He was also a cautionary tale having been separated from the Navy for taking too long to advance. The man rates a Purple Heart, but since he had Marines who did die in that battle, he refuses to wear it. Not enough promotable material to advance. That was a pretty big controversy at the time, and the exact position I did not want to be in. Under usual circumstances I would have left the Navy before the Navy left me, but because of the Uniform Code of Military Justice, it becomes a bit trickier to quit a job before being dismissed.

26 Sept 2020
Day 222

So, I've been pretty busy trying to transcribe all of these journal entries into Google Docs. Progress is coming along nicely, and it's a little fun to read what I was going through at any given time throughout the deployment. In a way, the mission was accomplished.

I am, however, tickled by how much I prefer to transcribe entries with just one day compared to multiple days' worth per entry. This is funny because every day gets its own page anyway so it shouldn't matter, but whatever.

It was a good day full of achievement and wonder. I was able to successfully coordinate the retrieval of HN Gunning's luggage. I thought it was good to be of use in a world where nothing is asked of me.

So there I was, talking on Messenger with my boy, Darren Malanik, about his recent breakup with his first love when out of the blue my own first love from high school messaged me. My fingers turned to lead. It was a surreal feeling, I never expected to hear from her again, and was resigned into accepting that. She wrote to thank me for the letter I wrote to her parents.

Saori dropped off some goodies for me and included Journal #1. I really think I'm going to finish this project before I leave. Well, phase one at least.

Josiah likes to see what I eat for breakfast. We call around that time and eat our meals together. Atticus needs a man in the home.

Postscript: During my senior year of high school, I moved out of my home and into my girlfriend's house. It might sound like a dream situation, but it wasn't. To oversimplify the situation, I wasn't the best son to my dad, and he was no angel either. When Bill and Jane Duckert took me in, I fell into their debt for as long as I live. One day I was at the kitchen table with Bill, and I told him I absolutely loved Baraboo, my hometown, and could just be there forever. Bill, an engineer for the Wisconsin Department of Transportation, said that he agreed, but only for the entire state of Wisconsin. Because I remembered that conversation, I mailed him a patch I had been carrying with me. The girl I dated is extremely private, one of the few people who requested not to have their name in the book, but still thought enough about it to reach out and thank me. Was still bizarre to hear from her, but thankful she did it.

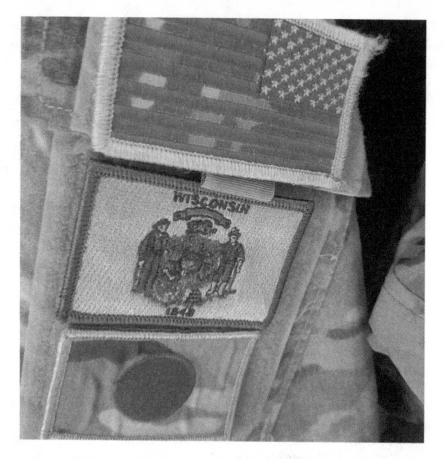

The patches, Wisconsin and Japan, were by no means authorized, but I snuck them in where I could. In order, this says where my heart was.

27 Sept 2020
Day 223

Wow, I am tired. I have spent most of my day in front of my computer. What started as a 0230 wake-up call, I laid in bed thinking for about an hour. There is something to be said about building a shelter for a rainy day. Maybe in other terms, to cover my six. Whatever; now is not the time to be cryptic.

I was thinking about possible jobs that'd keep me in Sasebo, but out of the Navy. Eventually I got out of bed and opened my laptop. An email from October 2019 that was never replied to, but always saved, was from Troops to Teachers. They were asking for a status update. Today I finally had that answer. I wrote my academic accomplishments and my goals saying I was a resident of Wisconsin, but my goal was to not only work in DODEA, but in Sasebo specifically. On top of that, I wrote to the DODEA Pacific-East region expressing interest. Getting my foot in the door, etc.

The deployment made me realize I can be separated from my family for the greater good of their welfare. Who knows, it's Sunday, no one is at work.

Had another long call with Brandon Schram. It's so nice to talk to an old friend. If only the rest of the old guard or a greatest hits guest list came back.

Knocked out 32 pages of transcribing today. At 11-point size font, I'm really building the document up. Took a three-hour nap. I'm very sore.

Postscript: I was sore from doing the bare minimum of exercising in my barracks room. Technically it was a suite of sorts. There were two bedrooms that led into a main entry room. From the entry room there was a sink and microwave, and next to it was a toilet/ shower room, and in the next room was another sink, I'm guessing more for morning beautification. In my situation, one bedroom was for sleeping, and the next bedroom was my gym and library. Because I was there for only 14 days, I did not do any interior decorating. Deciding what I was going to do after the Navy weighed heavily on my mind. If only I was one paygrade higher, I would be able to retire. This was not promised though, and I had to start making plans. I was due to leave my current command in April 2022 and wanted to make sure I was as ready as possible for a seamless transition.

28 Sept 2020
Day 224

Almost halfway there. This is night six I think, and the days are just drifting along. I think I'm starting to get out of jet-lag mode and experience the beginnings of a normal sleep schedule. Without aid of an alarm clock, I was out of bed by 0400. It helps when you fall asleep by 2130. This is particularly good because this is exactly what I predicted would happen when I got back to Sasebo. With 6.5 hours of sleep, I don't need to press snooze.

After waking up I was suddenly very focused and started to transcribe. By lunch I had completed Volume #1 of transcription. That was a day or two ahead of schedule. I'm at day 180 now, and if I work really hard, I will have become caught up by maybe tomorrow. That, to me, would have put me months ahead of where I was projecting this would end. Maybe quarantine does have its benefits after all.

After lunch I tried to fall asleep for a bit, but not without watching the Packer highlights. They beat the Saints 37-30. Without fail, Brandon Schram called shortly afterwards, but I couldn't stay mad, it was funny. That's the kind of guy he is. When I did get out of bed, I never did fall asleep, I logged into the Law School Admission Council website for the first time in like four years. There is an LSAT available in Tokyo in April 2021. I shot a message to Saori. She seemed supportive. Haven't really talked too much about the costs though.

Camp Rastall is going to have many hard discussions over the next few weeks.

Postscript: Preparing for a final descent out of the Navy took up a lot of my time. My thoughts were running wild, and this was prime research time while I was all by myself. Law school will probably be a dream I'll forever have, but as long as non-lawyers keep getting elected to government positions, the more hope I have that law school isn't the answer. Brandon liked to call me while I napped. Not like he knew when that was happening; he just wasn't one to nap while I decided to have a third child because I knew it extended the napping routine out at least another four years.

29 Sept 2020
Day 225

Another productive day despite being locked up. I never appreciated going to bed early so you can get up early as much as I have since my return to Sasebo. In the early morning, it's like the night still; how it's quiet and only the real dedicated are awake. Either you are still awake from the day before at 0400, or you're up early ready to tackle the day and wake up the birds.

For me though, I just wake up and roll out of bed. Of course, when I'm home in Arita the plan to start my day will be a little more elaborate than that by way of prepping clothes, food, bike, and to make sure I'm clear of distractions. How will I handle the smallest bit of adversity? I expect to now overcome it. Given my journey and the lessons gathered these 225 days, I should have the toolset to see a problem and adequately deal with it.

Hell yes, I'm excited to start the rest of my life and I want the rest of my life to start as soon as possible.

While transcribing, I write 30 to 40 pages a day. My style has not changed at all during the time I've been away. It surprises me that I didn't get, well, creative.

Saori thinks we are being released on Wednesday the 7th next week, but really it's the 6th. May I surprise her fittingly, like with flowers and stuff? We will see. But in the meantime, gotta be cool, calm, and collected.

Postscript: This was the second most time-consuming part of my thoughts while in ROM, what will my introduction back to society be like? How will I handle controversy? Do my problems minimize, or will they compound? I was worried about how I was going to behave, but more importantly react to everything. I wanted to think my conversations with LT Scott Byrd and everyone else have matured me and gotten me to a better position, but there is also a big difference between theory and application. I wasn't sure, and it had me concerned.

30 Sept 2020
Day 226

What I did today was be incredibly productive. So much so I was sleeping by 2130, again. Another theory is that I had spent too much time in front of my computer screen. Either way, it was a day of accomplishment.

I am now officially caught up with transcribing. After penning this entry, I will be immediately logging it into the computer, and that's a cool feeling.

Now I'm indexing everyone's name. Scrolling those 115+ pages, looking for names and citing them in the back is a daunting task. Actually, it's a joy compared to the content I'll have to review and revise on my next round of editing. This is such a tall order; I reached out to a professional editor I met before I left, Ms. Tori. We had an initial conversation, I shared the document on Gmail, and she said she'd look at it tomorrow. Hopefully she'll see the potential.

A title has been decided, *The Whiskey Journal: Definitely Not a Role III MMU Publication.* The subtitle is a callback to what I would put on each issue of *The Thirsty Camel.* It is a nod to those who I shared my life with in Whiskey Rotation.

Mrs. Rastall sent two big bags of grapes. That woman sure knows how to love me long time. She, of course, is getting the most citations I've noticed.

Tried to watch a documentary called *Netflix versus the World*, but I fell asleep. It was good and will finish when I wake up. Wrote a Letter of Authorization and Recommendation for Yani. It's for her commissioning package. I pretended to be the Officer in Charge of Sasebo as she requested, and he will review and sign later.

Postscript: To think that this was only 115 pages at one time! Even more impressive to me was how long it took to transcribe everything. That is a mark of dedication. I did not know exactly where I wanted this to go, but I knew I wanted to bring it somewhere. Tori was the first professional editor I ever met, and I was thankful for her guidance at this point in the process. The "Definitely Not a Role III MMU Publication" was my cheeky way of staying out of a legal spat with the United States Government and Department of the Navy. There is no blessing for this publication. I was too low on the totem pole to know anything important anyway. Plus, this publication had nothing to do with mission and strategy. The Taliban can suck it for all I care.

2 Oct 2020
Day 227 & 228

For a guy who is trapped in his room, there is plenty to unpack. There is plenty to talk about. A great deal of this is through the power and utility of the Internet.

Yesterday I reached out to an old UW-Green Bay friend, Danielle Behrle, who has started a beautiful family through marriage and now is Danielle LaCrosse. Because of social media, I've kept tabs on her, and knew she was a graphic designer.

It's an art and skill I've always admired and respected. Art class was never an "easy A" for me, in fact it was dreaded, and once I entered high school where I could choose my elective classes, I never set foot in the art department during the entire four years at Baraboo High School. Throw in computer integration, and it's game over. With that, I recognize it has its place and value in the market. My lack of familiarity does not diminish my appreciation for anyone who can excel in this field.

Anyway, Danielle didn't need much convincing to be onboard with the project. Since we're talking about outsourced talent to help make this experiment a reality, I heard back from my editor per say, Ms. Tori. She raised some good points with her questions.

Is this a piece for mass distribution or a record of my day? The editing will be different. After this I will be responding to her to essentially explain the first step is to make this a historical record that will one day be used for readers to know what my time was like. I also want to use it as source material for other projects, like my screenplay, where I will feel more comfortable taking more creative license on certain aspects.

This is all very exciting, and I look forward to putting in the work. In a way it helps to add two other people to the project because the extra pressure keeps me engaged. It's harder to slough off the work when others are expecting you to produce.

Josiah is at his first camping outing with the Cub Scouts. He's part of the Lion Den. Saori sent some pictures and I'm super proud of him. Next weekend he is doing it again where I plan to join him.

Called my mom yesterday. She was extra-saucy, but I think some of that is my inability to explain the future plans for myself and the family. I think in her mind I have less than eight years until retirement, and only a fool would leave a job so close to the end. She is not wrong, but there's just more to it than that. I keep adding sticks into the fire, and I don't know when to pull them out and make a decision. How fortified can I build my shelter for the rainy day that is either retirement or separation?

News is reporting President Trump now has COVID. If he gets criticized for hogging the attention away from Biden, then I applaud the brilliant strategy. Have to do some Scouting training now. Fun times.

Postscript: When I started my first business, the "Sconnie Sailor Moving Company," the funniest part was the thrill of having to learn something on my own or walk away from it knowing it was your fault. The triumphs and failures rest upon your shoulders. To understand there was more to a business than simply moving couches. For example, I never tried book-keeping before. That was a big step, but it was exciting to learn and become competent. Writing this book was no different; this is my next frontier, and I wanted to surround myself with people who knew more than me. Their feedback and assistance really helped push this along.

3 Oct 2020
Day 229

Now I'm starting to get anxious. The day is coming where I get to leave, and it's right around the corner. This leaves me very conflicted. Part of me is feeling apprehensive actually.

Sort of like that day in 8th grade when the class went to Noah's Ark waterpark in Wisconsin Dells. Not the time when I was drowning in the wave pool and the lifeguard had to jump in to save me despite wearing floaties on my arms; that's a different story. No, this story was about the vertical-drop ride called the "Point of No Return." How I was on the top, after climbing all those stairs and when I reached the summit, just dragged my feet to get in and get it all over with. It took my friend Michael-Paul, who finally looked me in the eyes to tell me that my crush at the time, Kate, was waiting and watching for me to go down. I saddled up and immediately conquered my fear to finish my journey.

Again, lots of time in front of a computer screen. Did most of the Cub Scout training, but there seemed to be a technical difficulty before I could completely finish.

I received an email from the Troops to Teachers Wisconsin representative. Essentially, a direct pipeline to DODEA is not an option, but I did ask what I can do in the interim to obtain Wisconsin licensure to teach. I should hear back next week.

Wrote an email to Greg Fall about my life of chess.

Although I did some editing, I was nicely interrupted by Brandon Schram. Josiah came back from his campout and I received reports that he was a well-behaved boy. Today he has his field day at his daycare, Atticus too. Saori is more fired up about it than they are. Ollie is looking cute as ever.

Postscript: The field days at the daycare are always a big deal. A lot of planning goes into them, and the preparation takes weeks or even months. In the military the term "field day" means you are cleaning. In this context, it's sports day and presentations for parents. In most ways I get it, a great killer of time throughout the day for kids to do that eventually leads up to something. Saori is all about them. I on the other hand now understand why there were so few band and choir concerts throughout the year because, as a parent, some of this stuff can be hard to sit through. That's not the Japanese way though, where encroaching on someone else's liberty and pride is possibly the #1 cultural sin. If you ever watch television in Japan, you'll know what I'm talking about.

4 Oct 2020
Day 230

Today was my last weekend away from home. For a Sunday I was surprised it was devoid of a nap, but I did however find time to relax by finally watching *Ford v Ferrari* (2019). The movie was enjoyable, but I don't know how it was some people's pick for the best movie of the year. I thought it didn't explain enough actually, like how Christian Bale and Matt Damon's characters even knew one another.

Because I watch Joe Rogan Experience clips on YouTube, I was led to the HBO docu-series *McMillions*, (2020), and after one episode I was not disappointed.

Edited a lot of pages today, too. Fingers crossed that I will get that leg of the project done tomorrow. As I'm reading through everything, I'm realizing how many little stories I missed out on. The reason for that I think is because with more people involved in a story, I would have needed more paper and it would have violated my one-page per day quota. It's a sad fact some stories will be lost to history, and everything can't be recorded. Maybe I'll increase the bulk and add them up in the "second half." Will consult with the editor.

Josiah and Atticus were being brothers on the phone, chasing one another with swords taking full swings at one another. Then there was Ollie, sitting there just watching as mayhem was unfolding at Camp Rastall.

Splurged today and got pizza & wings. Tasha Dayton brought beer, chips and salsa too. She went way above and beyond.

Postscript: Tasha Dayton was my first and only bookkeeper to help me stand up Sconnie Sailor Moving Company. My idea was more successful than I thought it would be, and I couldn't keep up with demand. Something had to give, and since I could afford it, hired Tasha, and she had since become a friend. It was a lazy Sunday; I was almost free of this place and getting set to come home.

5 Oct 2020
Day 231

Ah yes, my final day of the deployment. Tomorrow I'm slatted to go home and be released from the Restriction of Movement, or ROM, status. I mentioned this before, but there have been plenty of false finishes ever since the Transfer of Authority ceremony. It has been the longest road back home I'd ever taken, and it's finally coming to an end.

My time on my final day still had to be occupied though, and this is what I did. All of my self-editing is caught up. After this entry and tomorrow's sign-off post, a total of 57,000 words was written across 119 pages in size 11 font. After some email exchanges with Ms. Tori, I learned a fair market price for editing is about $0.035 per word. Quick math, this a $2,000 project at least. This does not include me tacking on a second half of side stories for amplification of characters. A price like that makes me think, and I have to start asking permission from people like Saori to continue. It's stressful, but a good kind of stress. Almost like the night before Christmas.

I'm on a roll with *McMillions* (2020) and I have one episode to go. I think it has plateaued, but hopefully the finale will bring it home. *Tiger King* (2020) was more entertaining.

Started to clean my room too. I had to repack my seabag as well. I'm not going to say the place is trashed, but it needs some love. The best part was having to empty out my fridge, to include all of the liquids. I anticipate getting up tomorrow later than I ever have before.

Yeah, this is a surreal feeling, and I'm fortunate it's over. Still though, my thoughts are with the reservists still grinding, waiting to go home.

Postscript: The mention about the reservists needs some attention. As active duty, we were all back at our permanent duty stations. The reservists had to process out of being "called up." Because of the COVID restrictions, they had to trickle through the processing center in Norfolk, VA, instead of getting it all done within a day or two, it took weeks of them sitting in a Norfolk hotel. With that said, ROM *in the states was very different from my experience in Sasebo, but our per capita infection rate supported our decision to be as "inconvenienced" as we were. There were times I'd watch the American news about COVID and think it seemed like that scene in* Titanic *(1997) when the flooding starts breaking through the glass and the grand staircase gets destroyed. Sheer panic and dread. I was going home the next day, and half of my teammates were still in Norfolk. As much as I wanted to be in that foxhole with them and "suffer" alongside them until it was over; I had the chance to go home and I took it.*

6 Oct 2020
Home: Day 0

Home. The story is over and another begins. Only this time I'm looking forward to it even more so than ever before.

Getting out of the barracks seemed like it would never end, but of course it did. Brandon Wydra dropped my truck, Bearjeau, off at the barracks and I loaded all my things to head straight into the clinic. That was about 1300.

By that time the Packers had a demanding enough lead on the Falcons of Atlanta. When it was over, it was a 30-16 Monday Night Football win, and that only added to the day.

While at the clinic, there was plenty that changed but more that was familiar. That was a nice feeling. I made my rounds seeing people. Because I walked in with my deployment uniform, I automatically had a talking point. My last stop was Master Chief Branch's office before I picked up mail and flowers.

I drove straight to the boys' daycare. Josey was already at swimming lessons, but Atticus ran into my arms and wouldn't let go. We walked home holding hands the entire way. It was a joy to meet Oliver for the first time. He's so far a very well-behaved baby.

Saori came home and was only half-surprised to see me. She of course sniffed it out that I was trying to surprise her. We walked to pick Josiah up and he wouldn't let me go either.

The first supper was yakiniku. It really hit the spot. I set up my new scale and clocked in at 304lb. After eight months I was hoping for a little more progress, but it's in the right direction.

The boys can almost wash themselves, and we read two books before bedtime. They were asleep by 2100.

Postscript: With the exception of Josiah and Atticus, I felt like how Bilbo may have felt coming back to the Shire. Everything is as it was. There was some fanfare at the clinic, many new faces, but there was no hero's parade. Why would there be? I volunteered for an easy deployment and came home. It was back to work. Back to reality, and I was excited for the next chapter.

Afterword

At the end, I continue to be torn in regard to my feelings on my time with Whiskey Rotation. Did I have a good time? No, I absolutely did not. Did I learn anything? What I learned was immeasurable. Would I do it again? It's funny to me how fast I was to volunteer and would think long and hard before I did it again.

My deployment was not in vain. After coming back to Branch Health Clinic Sasebo, I was named the Enlisted Watchbill Coordinator, a job I wanted for the last two years, and a position I was the assistant for during the last five years. My leadership believed that I was ready, and I would like to think they were correct. Then there was my selection as the Leading Petty Officer of Ancillary Services. This came as a surprise because I was competing against an E-6, and with seniority comes first preference when it comes to these kinds of selections. That was in January, but the icing of the cake was in March 2021 when it was my turn to be meritoriously promoted to First Class Petty Officer.

It was a long time coming. I would like to think that the deployment was the icing of the cake, but really it was the cake to put me over the hump for promotion. After eight years as Second Class Petty Officer, it felt surreal because I honestly believed that the day I would add another chevron to my rank was never going to happen. I now solidified myself to stay in the Navy until I am eligible to retire at 20 years of service.

I cried like a small child. They were tears of joy, of relief, and thanks for those who helped me along the way. The list is long of people who assisted me to get to where I am, and throughout these pages I hope to have drawn a fair enough outline as to how unconventional my road was. I had a lot of help from many different people, and I am thankful for their guidance, mentorship, oversight, invisible hand, and steadfast belief in me.

From the time I left Japan to when I returned, I lost an incredible five pounds. That is almost impossible. Some people actually pulled me aside when I came back and said, "Bro, why are you still fat?" It was a fair question, and one I worked through the entire time I was gone. There are the obvious excuses that no gym was open, fun was secured, and COVID, but that is exactly what that is, excuses. I was building a mindset that put me in the best position possible. When I came home, I lost 30 pounds relatively quickly. Then I strained my calf, and then warts grew on my foot hobbling me to the point of inactivity. Again excuses, and when I gained all that weight back, I realized a couple of things about myself.

First, there is the holy triad of weight loss: diet, exercise, and sleep. If any one of those three is missing you're going to have adverse results. I may think I'm eating like a rabbit, but the truth is I'm probably not, and that is why I need to exercise. The sleep prong is incredibly important too, because if I go to bed early, I can get up early and begin my day. I was right about the 6.5 hours of sleep too and have tried to live up to something I read regarding snooze buttons, "Why would I press snooze and fail at the first task of the day?" With proper sleep it eliminates the need for snooze. After recovering from getting hurt, I lost the weight again, and this time I continue that trend.

I still read often, and I find it important to read from different perspectives. No one book will have all the answers, but some books will speak to you differently than others. The only way to find out is to open them and find out for yourself. Reading opens doors, and it remains the single biggest talking point I can refer to when asked about self-improvement. As for my own writings that were mentioned, they are currently shelved and I hope to revisit them another day. Maybe *Opie & The Foreman* can be a children's book series (looking for the right illustrator. Is Bill Watterson looking for work?). The screenplay is queued after I finish my MBA and next book titled, *So There I Was: A Sailor's Sea Stories For Entry-Level Success.*

Lastly, there is the awareness that you need to do two things. You need to forgive yourself for your shortcomings, and you must extend your timeline out further than you are comfortable with. I still carry a lot of guilt and shame from my experiences with Whiskey, and most things everyone else may have forgotten, but it hangs on me. Once I'm able to shake from those shackles, I might be able to appreciate my time just that much more and look back upon what I accomplished with that much more pride. Secondly, by extending the timeline, I'm able to be comfortable with my progress and see a trend a lot more clearly. It's okay to lose "only" a pound a week provided it's still a lost pound. Not every workout will be a winner, not every trip to the scale will tell you what you want to read. Across time, given a long enough sample, it will though. That is something to be proud about.

My journey was memorable, and usually for all the wrong reasons. It had plenty of down moments, but they might have been teaching moments, and that is what I desperately needed at that time. There were plenty of teachers along the way. Did I accomplish everything I wanted to? No, I did not, but other things popped up in their place. I was never bored. I was only limited by my own complacency, and that was on me. Before I left, I wanted to learn Japanese, write a book, draft a screenplay, and lose 90 pounds. Of those goals, I partially completed one, and you are experiencing that product now. Much of my journey was an investment. Those who produce are rewarded, and I learned a lot about delayed satisfaction on this journey. Just because it is rated, or earned, or expected, or wanted, doesn't mean it'll come immediately. Much of my work came at the back end in the form of my evaluation, certificates, and even later my LPO role and eventual meritorious promotion. Had I been given so much up front, I am not sure if the real lessons would have been either taught or learned.

Abraham Lincoln wrote many of his speeches with the Declaration of Independence in mind. Much of what I wrote and how I thought was based off *A River Runs Through It.* Not exactly a 1:1 metaphor, but there was so much I thought about in terms of that movie and its narrator that I couldn't shake it the entire time I was away. Maybe a more relevant character might have been Jay Gatsby. What green light was I chasing, and did I ever capture it? I might have been involved in so much and extended myself, but at the end of the day, I felt pretty lonely, fixated on believing I wanted only one thing, and missing out on the beauty of everything else. Months after I returned, my pharmacist, Lieutenant Commander Sagrado, who was also at the Role III in another rotation, genuinely asked me how I felt about the deployment. The best answer I could muster was "doubt." I had no idea if what I was doing was worth it, and I believe that can be seen in these pages.

Things I purposely left out could be found in other sources such as the history of the Role III hospital in Kandahar and the layout of the base and the types of missions we accomplished. I tried to not put words in other people's mouths and limited my speculation on why people behaved how they did. I tried to look more inward and work through why I thought how I did, and my responses to certain stimuli. It really was a personal journey, one I am glad I could go on this ride. It would not age well mentioning the fall of Kabul to the Taliban less than a year after I left, but I will say that I'm glad to have been a part of a larger picture. COVID-19 changed everything and my experience at the Role III was so different than anyone else I met who served on previous rotations. There is something to be said about closing the longest-serving Navy combat hospital, and that is a piece of history I look forward to sharing as time moves on.

Because of this deployment, I will be able to retire from the Navy with at least 20 years of service. I look forward to one day donning a Veterans of Foreign Wars cap and marching with pride in parades of my hometown. I know I was part of something important, both from a historical perspective and personal experience. One day I'll believe what I did was just as much of a contribution to the preservation of freedom as others who did "real deployments." One day I won't be haunted by mistakes, and one day I will go home believing I did everything I could have done.

Stillness Is the Key Inscriptions

Referring to Day 213 & 214 written on September 18th, 2020, the following are the inscriptions from HM1 Wilson's book *Stillness is the Key*. For me, it will not be the challenge coins, the patches, or the t-shirts that will stay with me. This book, and the words written by as many people as I could find in the final days, will remain on my workbench for the rest of my days. Apologies to the Guam, mainland Japan, and Okinawa folks, but you all did get to leave early after all.

No message is placed in any particular order. They are all precious and meaningful to me. Thank you.

Cal,
There is no doubt that you'll do great things when the time is right. When things get tough, remember all of our talks.
1. [redacted].
2. In the military, if it doesn't make sense, then in fact that makes sense. Think from your heart, brother, always take care of others, and the rest will fall in place. Stay focused and take life one step at a time. I hope to see you again. - Jake (Wilson)

Cal Rastall,
Success comes with 3 things: compassion, confidence, and competence. (you spelled it right!) Keep these in mind with a positive attitude and it will take you wherever you want. Stay golden Pony Boy! - David Woolen

Cal,
You made the deployment a much brighter place! Your personality and sense of humor, not to mention your writing prowess, will be something I will always remember. Take care! - LCDR John Stewart

Thanks for the good jokes! Have a great life and good luck. - CDR Shaieb

HM1 (not a typing mistake),
Focus on the things that you can control and don't forget to invite us to the governor's mansion. Stay motivated! - CDR (Vince) Deguzman

HM2,
Continue to strive for greatness, but not at the expense of your sanity. All the best! - HM1 (Michael) LaPenna

Be natural and yourself, and this glittery flattery will be as the passing breeze at the sea on a warm summer day. - HM1 Wilson (again)

Cal,
It was good working with you and I wish you and your family all the best.
- Al Terrell

Rastall,
I was trying to think of something really cool to say but wanted it to be simple. So I'll share a favorite parting quote, "Be well, do good things, and stay in touch." - LT (Kevin) Veatch
P.S. If you find yourself in KY, find me, I'll buy first round!

"Great Serving" the last Roto with you brother!! Stay solid. - HM2 (Chris) Parchmon

A wise man told me once, FUCK YOU! He actually was a wise guy. Knowing the difference is the key. Have fun, fart, and grow old. See you later! You Rock! - LCDR Chris Van Pelt

A bird in the hand is worth TWO in the bush. Remembering this will keep you young and happy for life. Be well my cheese-headed friend. - HM2 (Wilbon) Robinson

Cal,
You will always be someone I remember on this deployment. I will never forget the "Ari Gold" *Thirsty Camel* article you wrote. My family loved it, and so did I. Stay in touch big guy! - HM2 (Nick) Slagle

Hafa Adai, from Guam - (Claudine) Bansil

Rastall,
It has been great to work with you! I appreciate your good attitude every time I woke you for meds...after I told you I was all set for the night. Your newsletter was a highlight of deployment. Good luck! - LT (Michele) Taylor

HM2,
I don't even know where to begin with my long list of thank yous. I'll start with my appreciation of all your hard work and thoughtfulness in regard to the newsletter and all the other projects you took on. It was a pleasure working with you and witnessing your growth as a leader and mentor - I think we all grew a lot together. I wish you well and know you

will be a great success whether it's in the Navy or the literary world. Please keep in touch. - LCDR (Kate) Fitz(gerald)

HM2,
Been a pleasure bro! Keep up the solid work and "thank you." v/r HMCS (Cameron Wink)

18Sep20
HM2 Rastall,
You are a most unique and gifted individual. Every interaction with you on this deployment was a distinct honor. I picked this chapter as there is too much escapism, but I'm confident you'll resist it. Remember that the opposite of depression is purpose–use this to your advantage. Never hesitate to contact me as a mentor. - D.E. Kahler, DO

Our deepest fear is not that we are inadequate. Our deepest fear is that we are powerful beyond measure. It is our light, not our darkness that most frightens us…

Rastall, Do big things, never quit. It was a pleasure. -The LT (Scott) Byrd

Rascal,
It's been a pleasure serving with you. Think of me whenever you hear the Austrian Band, AC-DC. -CDR Phil Self aka PMS

HM2,
What can be said to a man of such talent and wonderful character! All the best to you. Family and I hope to meet you and them together some day! Best, COT (CDR John Mayberry)

HM2,
It was so nice meeting you on this deployment! I wish you all the best! - The Kidd LT (Sherry Kidd)

HM2,
It was great getting to know you and work with you on this deployment. I hope that you have a long and great career in the Navy. Really enjoyed your "editorial." All the best! - CDR (Jud) Nash

Cal,
Don't change anything about you. I love your honesty and frankness; the world could use more of that these days. Wish you well in your life. - Blades, Joanna

RAY-STALL!
Great to know you man. Hope to work with you one day again. If only there was a JJ Rah-stall starting at Wisconsin in 19 years.... - J(eff) Klinger

Cal (HM2),
Thank you for being you man. Always enjoyed our discussions AND I look forward to reading more of that screenplay. You know how to get in touch! Do great things. "Those who dare to fail miserably, can achieve greatly."-JFK -Gibby (Jonathan Gibford)

HM2,
Thanks for keeping things light and all you did behind the scenes for the rotation. It is obvious that you are destined for great things. Keep cultivating your creativity. - DFA (Director For Administration)

HM2,
A pleasure working with you! Always kind, attentive and hardworking. Enjoy the family. -Carmen Davis

HM2,
Thank you for some wonderful conversations and all you did for our roto and our country. You are an amazing person and I am honored to know you. -Sam Reeder

HM2,
It has been a pleasure knowing you. I will miss the Camel Toe Issue. It made some light of stressful individuals. Best of luck with all you do in the future. I'm certain you will succeed in anything you do. Let me know if there is anything I can ever do for you. Take care, Tom v/r LCDR Warner

Be patient - Ho Vo

Cal,
It was great being deployed with you and reading your *Thirsty Camel.* Keep pushing - Jake (Kubil)

It's been an absolute pleasure working with you! Send me your screenplay as soon as it's finished! -HM2 (Wes) Alden

Rastall,
You are a man of very complex words. Future politician that I will vote for. Continue to do great things, and don't stop! You never know who else you are inspiring. -Jedi "that mothafucka" Rodriguez

Love you :) - (James) Writer

HM2,
You were able to bring humor and smiles to an otherwise not so funny experience. Thank you!! - LT (Ben) Wilcox

HM2,
It's been a pleasure working with you! I enjoyed our talks @ the pit! Good luck with your future endeavors! - Bernie

HM2,
It was great deploying with you. The newspaper thing brought a lot of humor and smiles! -HM2 (Johnpatrick) Arboleda

Cal,
Looking forward to running into you again just like I looked forward to the next issue of *The Thirsty Camel.* - (Robert) [redacted]

HM2,
Thanks for the laughs. Glad to have met you. -LT (Greg) Downey

Can't wait to read the first copy of your book! -LT W (Geneva Wilson)

Catch ya on the flipside!!!!!!!!!!!!!!!!!!! -MA2 (Robert) Krombach

HM2,
Pleasure meeting you and working with you. Wish you the best in all your future Navy adventures! -LT (Lori) Quinn

Special Thanks

Normally reserved for my family, I would like to personally thank the Navy for making this process to publication about twice as long as it could have been. In seriousness, the US Navy has given me essentially every good thing that has come in my life, and I'm happy to be employed by them. After all, a bitching Sailor is a happy Sailor (it means they still have hope!). My wife, who was patient with me when I had to escape to write, and my boys, who gave me something to write for. Josiah, Atticus and Oliver, remember this and know it well, Papa loves you, and he knows his Navy salary isn't going to pay for your college, so this is him trying to do something about that. To the publisher who took a chance on me, Angela Hoy, and her entire team who judo'd this into a reality. My everlasting gratitude is extended to you all for keeping me out of trouble. To my longtime friend Danielle LaCrosse who was instrumental in the cover design and Todd Engel who tied it all together. The list could go on, but not without explicitly acknowledging Kathryn Silva for brushing up the language and making it tight. To everyone who kept me on the hook to push through this so that it could see the light of day, you should know who you are and I thank you, too.

CPSIA information can be obtained
at www.ICGtesting.com
Printed in the USA
LVHW101605170922
728624LV00006B/355